Gluten-Free & Dairy-Free Meal Prep Cookbook

Easy and Satisfying Recipes without Gluten or Dairy | Save Time, Lose Weight and Improve Health | 30-Day Meal Plan

Kelly Hearner

Table of contents

Introduction

Cooking meals when you are on a specific diet restriction become challenging, especially on busy weekdays.

So, how can you get ahead of this?

The ideal solution for you is meal prepping. Meal prepping can make a significant difference in your healthy lifestyle without any stress home cooking. The focus of this e-book is on gluten-free meals.

Meal prepping gives you the charge of your own meals by giving you a head start on your breakfast, lunch, and dinners, even desserts as well. You just need to take some time on Sunday to get everything together, and in the next week, you will have tasty and healthy meals ready to go. Here's what you will find in the 30-Days gluten-free meal plan:

- Ready to go meals
- Make head meals
- Slow cooker meals
- Quick Salads
- No-cook meals
- Freezable meals
- No-Bake desserts

And, all are fresh, healthy, 100% delicious!

Chapter 1: Understanding the Gluten-Free Diet

What is gluten?

Gluten, a family of protein, is found in grains like ryes, wheat, and spelt are gluten-containing grains. Gluten is responsible for forming a sticky network or adding a glue-like consistency in the foods like in dough for loaves of bread, cookies, etc. Gluten adds elasticity into the dough, gives the bread to rise when baked, and delivers it a satisfying texture.

Gluten is made up of two main proteins that are gliadin and glutenin. Among these two proteins, glutenin has most of the adverse effects on health. Although most of the people are gluten tolerant but it can cause harmful effects for the people with certain conditions, which includes people suffering from gluten sensitivity, celiac diseases, wheat allergies, etc.

The most common symptom of gluten intolerance is digestion discomfort. There could be other reasons for this discomfort as well. If you think you have digestive comfort, ask your doctor to check you for celiac disease first. If the test comes out positive, consult your doctor first before trying the gluten-free diet. But, if you don't have celiac diseases, the best way to figure out if you are gluten intolerance is through strictly follow a gluten-free diet for few weeks. Then introduce the gluten back into your diet and see if its symptoms are improving or not.

What foods contains gluten?

Starting with a gluten-free diet can be challenging at the start. You will have to shift on eating whole foods as they are naturally gluten-free. Along with the changes in the diet, you will have to start reading food labels on everything you are purchasing in the grocery store or when eating out. The following foods are the most common sources of gluten.

Grains

- Wheat
- Rye
- Spelt
- Bread
- Pasta
- Cereal
- Crackers

- Cake
- Cookies
- Pastries
- All sort of wheat-based baked foods

Fruits and Vegetables

- Canned vegetables and fruits
- Frozen vegetables and fruits
- Dried fruits
- Pre-chopped vegetables and fruits

Proteins

- Processed meals like bacon, salami, pepperoni and hot dogs
- Cold cuts meats
- Breaded meat, fish or poultry
- Seitan

Dairy Products

- Flavored milks
- Flavored yogurts
- Processed cheese product
- Cheese sauces
- Spreads
- Malted milk drinks

Fats and Oils

- Cooking sprays
- Oils with added spices and flavors

Beverages

- Premade smoothies
- All beverages with added flavoring
- Distilled liquor
- Vodka
- Whiskey
- Gin

Sauces and condiments

- Wheat-based soy sauce
- Wheat-based teriyaki sauce
- Malt vinegar

The gluten-free diet for weight loss

Apart from people suffering from celiac diseases, many people have started following a gluten-free diet for dropping extra pounds of weight. And, the results have been magical. So instead of eating carefully, doing plenty of exercises, take a diet devoid of gluten and wheat. Here are some strategies to lose weight when you are on a gluten-free diet.

1. Avoid processed gluten-free foods

You will need to steer clear from wheat and gluten-free processed foods. There are some grain-free gluten-free products like gluten-free cake mixes, snacks, cookies, pizza, and bread, but they actually have higher calories than their wheat-based versions. So, don't take the label of gluten-free food products as "calorie-free."

2. Count your calories

Just like you used to count calories on the non-gluten-free diet, you have keep continuing this when you go gluten-free. You will find drop in your weight effortlessly as gluten-free diet curb the cravings and appetite. As a result, you eat fewer calories. However, you need to keep check on your calorie intake to keep your weight loss ball rolling.

3. Eat low-carb or Paleo also

Along with cutting the carbs and gluten from the wheat, giving up every high-carb food is best for weight loss on a gluten-free diet. However, make sure you are still consuming fiber, valuable vitamins, and other nutrients as well to meet your dietary requirements.

4. Don't forget to exercise

Exercise is the most important tip of all for losing weight on a gluten-free diet. Eliminating the gluten and wheat may help in losing weight more quickly, but if you want to speed things up, you are going to need to break a sweat. Hitting the gym and doing exercise can help in losing even more fat. So, along with following the gluten-free diet to the T, you need to make some time for some healthy physical activities as well.

Chapter2: Why Meal Prep?

The benefits of meal prep

You love cooking, but you need to have some motivation to use your kitchen for homemade meals. Cooking food on your own is the best way to boost your health and have more control over what food you're consuming. The food you eat assimilates into your bodies and becomes part of your blood, cells, and even thoughts and feelings. Learning to cook high-quality food for yourself and those you love changes everything in life; home cooking ultimately allows the ability to manage your food allergies and sensitivities, as well as portion sizes. Also, home cooking nourishes you, mind, body, and soul. When you start to put our energy into making food, you ultimately put that energy back into ourselves. Eating home-cooked meals five or more days a week is even associated with a longer life.

However, home cooking is an overwhelming chore. You have prep ingredients for food, do the dishes, and then cleaning kitchen utensils after each round of cooking. Daunting, isn't it? But not anymore! What if you can have to do cooking only once for a week-long meal. Yes, you can do this with meal prepping. Meal prepping is a blessing in disguise for new cooks and busy professionals who love home cooking or are focused on eating healthy foods at home. Meal prepping is more than that.

- Bulk cooking saves you

One of the personal favorite ways to cook at home on a limited timeframe is to use the idea of "freezer cooking." It requires cooking for one or two days a month and then freezing them to feed the family for the whole month. With frozen home-cooked foods, you can enjoy meals throughout the month. And, they will save you from the stress of cooking on busy days when you don't have much time to be in the kitchen. Even cooking ahead and that too in bulk is great if you are hosting a party or a grand family dinner.

- Total control on foods

When you cook your own meals or plan what to eat in advance, you get to be a total control freak, in a right way by gaining complete control of calories and macro balance. It ultimately reduces the usage of unnecessary ingredients like added sugar, salt, and fats, and you come to know exactly which ingredients and how much of each is going into our food. By this, meal prepping makes sure that you get the best quality meals with more fresh ingredients because you are selecting them on our own.

- Meal Prep is cheaper than eating out

Eating out is a tasty treat every once in a while, but it's also expensive. There are places where you can eat out cheap foods regularly, but that's living an unhealthy lifestyle. It is time to make a change in your life with a meal prepping restaurant styled food in your home kitchen. Firstly, cooking at home will probably save your money because you won't be ordering any lunch or dinner in a restaurant. And, you can pick your favorite meal prep recipes and make sure the ingredients used in them are fresh and organic and cook to the T. If you wish to save more money, you can plan your meal prep as per ingredients available on sales at the grocery stores.

- Cooking is therapeutic

Research has proven that activities involving the kitchen like cooking are a great stress reliever because they are considered an act of patience. Have you ever heard about culinary mindfulness, culinary therapy, and therapeutic cooking? These methods are practice to stabilize your mental health through the culinary. So, yes cooking at home plays an important role in improving your mental health. Along with patients, when you cook for your loved ones or just for yourself, you will always feel like you have accomplished something. Similarly, if you have anxiety or depression, you can treat it with your cooking activity at home, because doing this creative task create positive effects on your mind.

How do you meal prep and eat healthy?

Our lives are getting busy day by day and in this all the chaos of the world, what we do and eat for our meals effects our lives. Often, there won't be any choice for you but to take shortcuts when it comes to meal, but it will cost your life in the future. Of course, when there is so much going on in your life, you can't focus on cooking tasty meals thrice a day. But, cooking ahead meals can save your time and maintain your healthy lifestyle. Following are some simple cooking meal prepping tips that will make cooking way too simple for you.

1. Make a Plan

Firstly, you need to decide what you are going to cook and this will saves your energy and time you spend thinking about cooking for every meal. Plan all the recipes you want to prepare for the week or month and put together a grocery list by making a list of their ingredients. Don't go for variety as these recipes will not have common ingredients, and each meal will take a lot of cooking time. If you are new at meal prepping, it is better to start with two to three recipes per week.

2. Pick the right combination of recipes

So, I have been talking about saving time through meal prepping, but how you can achieve this? By cooking multiple foods at once. For example, you can roast vegetables along with the baking chicken in a sheet pan at the same time. It will speed things up in the kitchen. But at time, it can be tricky to figure out number of meals you should cook and their best combination for cooking. For this, your past meal prepping experiences will help you. So, check your last food calendar and then plan accordingly for the upcoming week or month.

3. Don't meal prep too many meals

At the beginning of your meal prep journey, focus on preparing one recipe at a time and make large batches of it. Then split it into individual portions that need to freeze and then eat the food over the next few months. Make-ahead your meal calendar and follow it religiously. It may happen that cooking a full week's worth of meals in a day may be stressful for you, so start with cooking twice a week.

4. Pick the right food container for storage

Your meal prepping activities will only be successful if you can maintain your meal freshness and delicious taste. In that, meal prep containers can help you a lot. When your food is ready to store, use airtight containers to store its portions. Heatproof glass container and stainless steel container about 3 to 5 inches in depth, and silicon baggies are great options for keeping your prepared foods fresh and crispy; avoid plastic utensils.

How long does food stay good when you are meal prep?

If you are making valiant efforts in your food prep and it's more than your weekly routine, so you also need to ensure that you store and reheat your foods in the right way. In this way, you can prevent your foods from any poison and harm to your health.

Although you can store your foods in the refrigerator, freezing these meals is a much better option. It means that just prepare a variety of nutritious dishes, store them in the freezer and then fix them as many times you want in the week or month. One essential detail to ensure your prepped food can be stored in the refrigerator is that it should be set at 40 degrees F or below.

Moreover, you also need to invest your time in organizing, dating, and labeling your ready meals. Through this, you will exactly know how long the dish last. Also, keep your meal fresh longer by wrapping each portion tightly in plastic wrap or aluminum foil because oxygen is a catalyst for food spoilage.

Some more valuable tips for storing foods are:

- Refrigerated foods go smelly after three to five days, so eat them accordingly.
- Salads and dishes that have seafood are best to refrigerate for up to five days
- Store cooked vegetables and meat for five days

Boiled eggs are good to eat for up to 1 week.

Chapter3: 30-Day Meal Plan

Day 1

Breakfast: Granola

Lunch: Chicken Mason Jar Salad

Dinner: Almond Butter Turkey Meatballs

Dessert: Matcha Coconut Tarts

Day 2

Breakfast: Granola

Lunch: Chicken Mason Jar Salad

Dinner: Almond Butter Turkey Meatballs

Dessert: Matcha Coconut Tarts

Day 3

Breakfast: Granola

Lunch: Roasted Tomatoes and Mushrooms

Dinner: Bean and Beef Slow-Cooked Chili

Dessert: Matcha Coconut Tarts

Day 4

Breakfast: Granola

Lunch: Roasted Tomatoes and Mushrooms

Dinner: Bean and Beef Slow-Cooked Chili

Dessert: Matcha Coconut Tarts

Day 5

Breakfast: Parsnip Hash Browns

Lunch: Tuna Salad Lettuce Wraps

Dinner: Orange Tofu Chickpea Bowls

Dessert: Blueberry Custard Pie

Day 6

Breakfast: Parsnip Hash Browns

Lunch: Tuna Salad Lettuce Wraps

Dinner: Shrimp Avocado Salad

Dessert: Blueberry Custard Pie

Day 7

Breakfast: Almond Cranberry Chocolate Granola Bars

Lunch: Thai Turkey Lettuce Wraps

Dinner: Lime Shrimp Zoodles

Dessert: Blueberry Custard Pie

Day 8

Breakfast: Almond Cranberry Chocolate Granola Bars

Lunch: Thai Turkey Lettuce Wraps

Dinner: Honey Sesame Chicken

Dessert: Blueberry Custard Pie

Day 9

Breakfast: Almond Cranberry Chocolate Granola Bars

Lunch: Stuffed Portobello Mushrooms

Dinner: Honey Sesame Chicken

Dessert: Collagen Brownie Cups

Day 10

Breakfast: Almond Cranberry Chocolate Granola Bars

Lunch: Tofu Stir Fry

Dinner: Lemon Butter Veggies and Sausage

Dessert: Collagen Brownie Cups

Day 11

Breakfast: Sausage Hash Brown Casserole

Lunch: Beef Ragu Pasta

Dinner: Lemon Butter Veggies and Sausage

Dessert: Collagen Brownie Cups

Day 12

Breakfast: Sausage Hash Brown Casserole

Lunch: Beef Ragu Pasta

Dinner: Quinoa and Black Bean Stuffed Peppers

Dessert: Collagen Brownie Cups

Day 13

Breakfast: Broccoli and Red Pepper Egg Muffins

Lunch: Cilantro Lime Chicken with Cauliflower Rice

Dinner: Honey Lemon Salmon and Broccolini

Dessert: Rice Crispy Treats

Day 14

Breakfast: Broccoli and Red Pepper Egg Muffins

Lunch: Cilantro Lime Chicken with Cauliflower Rice

Dinner: Honey Lemon Salmon and Broccolini

Dessert: Rice Crispy Treats

Day 15

Breakfast: Broccoli and Red Pepper Egg Muffins

Lunch: Sweet Potato, Lentil and Kale Salad

Dinner: Buffalo Chicken Casserole

Dessert: Rice Crispy Treats

Day 16

Breakfast: Broccoli and Red Pepper Egg Muffins

Lunch: Sweet Potato, Lentil and Kale Salad

Dinner: Buffalo Chicken Casserole

Dessert: Rice Crispy Treats

Day 17

Breakfast: Pancakes

Lunch: Steak and Garlic Roasted Potato

Dinner: Orange-Sage Pork Chops

Dessert: Chocolate Chia Pudding

Day 18

Breakfast: Pancakes

Lunch: Steak and Garlic Roasted Potato

Dinner: Burger and Veggie Bowls

Dessert: Chocolate Chia Pudding

Day 19

Breakfast: Breakfast Power Bowl

Lunch: Sweet Potato and Lentil Salads

Dinner: Grilled Vegetable and Black Bean Bowls

Dessert: Lime And Avocado Tart

Day 20

Breakfast: Breakfast Power Bowl

Lunch: Sweet Potato and Lentil Salads

Dinner: Grilled Vegetable and Black Bean Bowls

Dessert: Lime And Avocado Tart

Day 21

Breakfast: Turkey and Artichokes Breakfast Casserole

Lunch: Tuna and White Bean Salad

Dinner: Cod and Veggies

Dessert: Lime And Avocado Tart

Day 22

Breakfast: Turkey and Artichokes Breakfast Casserole

Lunch: Tuna and White Bean Salad

Dinner: Cashew Chicken

Dessert: Lime And Avocado Tart

Day 23

Breakfast: Turkey and Artichokes Breakfast Casserole

Lunch: Caprese Chicken Salad

Dinner: Garlic Peppered Steak

Dessert: Brownies

Day 24

Breakfast: Turkey and Artichokes Breakfast Casserole

Lunch: Caprese Chicken Salad

Dinner: Tuna Cakes

Dessert: Brownies

Day 25

Breakfast: Omelet Muffins

Lunch: Jalapeno Sliders

Dinner: Tuna Cakes

Dessert: Brownies

Day 26

Breakfast: Omelet Muffins

Lunch: Jalapeno Sliders

Dinner: Lemon Herb Chicken with Vegetables

Dessert: Brownies

Day 27

Breakfast: Omelet Muffins

Lunch: Chili Beef Pasta

Dinner: Lemon Herb Chicken with Vegetables

Dessert: Chocolate Almond Bark

Day 28

Breakfast: Omelet Muffins

Lunch: Chili Beef Pasta

Dinner: Pulled Pork Taco Bowl

Dessert: Chocolate Almond Bark

Day 29

Breakfast: Cinnamon Raisin Granola

Lunch: Moroccan Chickpea Quinoa Salad

Dinner: Pulled Pork Taco Bowl

Dessert: Chocolate Almond Bark

Day 30

Breakfast: Cinnamon Raisin Granola

Lunch: Moroccan Chickpea Quinoa Salad

Dinner: Salad with Chickpeas and Tuna

Dessert: Chocolate Almond Bark

Chapter 4: Breakfast and Brunch

Turkey and Artichokes Breakfast Casserole

Preparation time: 15 minutes
Cooking time: 60 minutes
Servings: 12

Ingredients:

- 1 1/2 pound ground turkey
- 2 green onion, sliced
- 1 medium green bell pepper, diced
- 14 ounces artichoke hearts, chopped
- 2 ½ cups fresh baby spinach
- 1/2 of a medium onion, peeled, diced
- 1/2 teaspoon cumin
- ¾ teaspoon ground black pepper
- 1/2 teaspoon oregano
- 1 teaspoon salt
- 1 teaspoon red chili powder
- 2 tablespoons avocado oil
- 16 eggs, beaten

Method:

1. Switch on the oven, then set it to 375 degrees F and let preheat.
2. Meanwhile, take a skillet pan, place it over medium heat, add oil and when hot, add onion and green bell pepper.
3. Then add turkey, season with cumin, black pepper, oregano, salt, and red chili powder, stir well and cook for 10 minutes until meat is thoroughly cooked and nicely browned.
4. Add 2 cups spinach into cooked meat, stir well and continue cooking for 2 minutes until spinach leaves have wilted.
5. Take a 9 by 13 inches casserole dish or twelve oven safe meal prep glass containers, spoon in the turkey-spinach mixture, spread it evenly, and then top with artichokes.
6. Beat the eggs, pour it over artichokes in the casserole, and then sprinkle with green onion and remaining spinach and bake the casserole for 45 minutes until thoroughly cooked.
7. For meal prepping, let casserole or containers cool completely, then cover the casserole well with aluminum foil or close the containers with lid and store in the refrigerator for up to five days or freeze for three months.
8. Reheat casserole in the microwave until hot and serve.

Nutrition Value:

- Calories: 184.7 Cal
- Fat: 11.7 g
- Carbs: 6.2 g
- Protein: 13.9 g
- Fiber: 2.5 g

Granola

Preparation time: 10 minutes
Cooking time: 20 minutes
Servings: 10

Ingredients:

- 1 cup raisins
- 3 cups rolled oats, old-fashioned
- 1 cup sliced almonds
- 1/2 teaspoon ground cinnamon
- 1/2 teaspoon salt
- 1/2 cup honey
- 1/2 cup olive oil

Method:

1. Switch on the oven, then set it to 300 degrees F, then place the baking rack in the middle of the oven and let preheat.
2. Place oil in a large bowl, whisk in cinnamon, salt, and honey until combined, then add almonds and oats and stir until well coated.
3. Take a rimmed baking sheet, line it with parchment paper, spoon oats mixture on it, then spread it in an even layer and bake for 20 minutes until granola is golden brown, stirring halfway through.
4. Sprinkle raisins on top of granola, press it lightly and then let the granola cool.
5. Break granola into small pieces, then transfer granola into an airtight container and store for up to one month at room temperature.
6. When ready to eat, add some of the granola in a bowl, pour in milk, top with berries and serve.

Nutrition Value:

- Calories: 322 Cal
- Fat: 17.1 g
- Carbs: 40.5 g
- Protein: 5.7 g
- Fiber: 4 g

Almond Cranberry Chocolate Granola Bars

Preparation time: 20 minutes
Cooking time: 25 minutes
Servings: 12

Ingredients:

- 1 1/2 cups rolled oats, old-fashioned
- 1/4 cup chocolate chips
- 3/4 cup sliced almonds
- 1/3 cup cranberries, dried
- 1/3 cup honey
- 1/8 teaspoon salt
- 2 tablespoons brown sugar
- 3 tablespoons butter, unsalted
- 1/2 teaspoon vanilla extract, unsweetened
- 2 tablespoons peanut butter

Method:

1. Switch on the oven, then set it to 325 degrees and let preheat.
2. Take a medium saucepan, place it over medium-low heat, add the butters, honey, sugar, salt, and vanilla, stir well until combined and cook for 5 minutes until the sugar has dissolved and butter has melted.
3. Meanwhile, place oats in a medium bowl, add almonds and stir until mixed.
4. Pour in prepared honey mixture, stir until well combined, and let the mixture stand at room temperature for 10 minutes.
5. Then add chocolate chips and cranberries and fold until just mixed.
6. Take a 9 by 9 inches casserole dish, line it with parchment sheet, spoon in prepared oats mixture, spread and firmly press into the pan by using the back of a glass and bake for 25 minutes until crunchy.
7. Let the granola cool in the pan on a wire rack, then cut into twelve bars and store in an airtight container for up to one week at room temperature or refrigerate for up to one month.

Nutrition Value:

- Calories: 190 Cal
- Fat: 13 g
- Carbs: 18 g
- Protein: 4 g
- Fiber: 5 g

Cinnamon Raisin Granola

Preparation time: 10 minutes
Cooking time: 30 minutes
Servings: 5

Ingredients:

- 1 cup shredded coconut, unsweetened
- 1/2 cup raisins
- 1 cup pumpkin seeds
- 1/2 cup chopped pecans
- 1 cup sunflower seeds
- 1/2 cup sliced almonds
- 1/4 teaspoon salt
- 1/2 teaspoon allspice
- 1 tablespoon cinnamon
- 1 teaspoon vanilla extract, unsweetened
- 2 tablespoons maple syrup
- 1/3 cup coconut oil
- 1/4 cup honey

Method:

1. Switch on the oven, then set it to 300 degrees F and let it preheat.
2. Meanwhile, place all the ingredients in a large bowl, except for vanilla, maple syrup, oil, and honey and stir until well mixed.
3. Take a saucepan, place it over low heat, add vanilla, maple syrup, oil, and honey, stir well and cook for 5 minutes until melted.
4. Meanwhile, take a 10 by 15 inches baking sheet and then line it with parchment paper.
5. Pour this mixture over granola mixture in the bowl and mix by hand until combined.
6. Transfer granola mixture onto the prepared baking sheet, spread it evenly, and bake for 25 minutes until golden brown, stirring halfway through.
7. Cool the granola on a wire rack and then break it into small pieces.
8. Transfer granola into an airtight container and then store for up to one month at room temperature.
9. When ready to eat, add some of the granola in a bowl, pour in milk, top with berries and serve.

Nutrition Value:

- Calories: 129.2 Cal
- Fat: 1 g
- Carbs: 31 g
- Protein: 1 g
- Fiber: 4.1 g

Broccoli and Red Pepper Egg Muffins

Preparation time: 10 minutes
Cooking time: 20 minutes
Servings: 8

Ingredients:

- 1/2 cup roasted red pepper, cored, diced
- 1/2 cup broccoli florets, riced
- 1/2 teaspoon ground black pepper
- 1/2 teaspoon salt
- 1/2 teaspoon garlic powder
- 1 tablespoon coconut milk, unsweetened
- 4 eggs
- 4 egg whites

Method:

1. Switch on the oven, then set it to 325 degrees F, and let it preheat.
2. Meanwhile, whisk the eggs and egg whites in a large bowl and then beat in black pepper, salt, garlic powder, and milk until combined.
3. Then add red pepper and riced broccoli and stir until mixed.
4. Take an eight cups muffin pan, grease its cups with oil, then evenly fill with prepared broccoli and red pepper mixture and bake for 20 minutes until eggs are set and muffins are firm in the center.
5. When done, take out muffins from the muffin pan and let cool on the wire rack.
6. For meal prep, wrap each muffin with aluminum foil and refrigerate for up to five days or freeze for up to one month.
7. When ready to eat, reheat the muffin in the microwave until hot and serve.

Nutrition Value:

- Calories: 73.7 Cal
- Fat: 4.8 g
- Carbs: 1.7 g
- Protein: 6.4 g
- Fiber: 0.6 g

Pancakes

Preparation time: 10 minutes
Cooking time: 12 minutes
Servings: 4

Ingredients:

- 1 cup coconut flour
- 1/4 cup coconut oil, melted
- 1 1/2 cups almond milk, unsweetened
- 8 eggs
- Strawberries, fresh, for topping

Method:

1. Place flour in a large bowl, add oil, milk, and eggs and beat until smooth batter comes together.
2. Take a skillet pan, place it over medium heat, grease it with oil and when hot, add 3 tablespoons of batter per pancake in it and cook the pancake for 3 minutes per side until nicely golden from both sides.
3. Cook more pancakes in the same manner until all the batter is used up.
4. Let pancakes cool, then divide them evenly between four ovenproof meal prep containers, stacking pancakes with wax paper in between, and add strawberries.
5. Cover the containers with lid and freeze for up to two months.
6. When ready to eat, reheat pancakes in the microwave for 2 minutes until hot and serve.

Nutrition Value:

- Calories: 375 Cal
- Fat: 27 g
- Carbs: 17 g
- Protein: 16 g
- Fiber: 5 g

Breakfast Power Bowl

Preparation time: 10 minutes
Cooking time: 0 minutes
Servings: 2

Ingredients:

- 1 cup shredded carrots
- 1/2 cup lentils, cooked
- 2 cups quinoa, cooked
- 1 medium avocado, peeled, pitted, thinly sliced
- 1 cup shredded red cabbage
- 1/2 teaspoon garlic powder
- 1/4 teaspoon cumin
- 6 eggs, hard-boiled

Method:

1. Place cooked quinoa in a large bowl, add lentils, sprinkle with cumin and garlic powder and stir until combined.
2. Take meal prep containers, fill them evenly with quinoa mixture, and then evenly add shredded carrots and cabbage.
3. Peel the boiled eggs, then cut each egg in half and place them on top with quinoa along with avocado slices.
4. Cover the containers with lid and store in the refrigerator for up to five days and serve when required.

Nutrition Value:

- Calories: 439 Cal
- Fat: 19 g
- Carbs: 44 g
- Protein: 23 g
- Fiber: 14 g

Sausage-Hash Brown Casserole

Preparation time: 10 minutes
Cooking time: 45 minutes
Servings: 6

Ingredients:

- 6 sausages, sliced
- 1 cup fresh spinach
- 4 cups shredded potatoes
- ½ teaspoon ground black pepper
- 2/3 teaspoon salt
- 1 1/3 cup egg whites
- 6 eggs

Method:

1. Switch on the oven, then set it to 350 degrees F and let preheat.
2. Meanwhile, take a skillet pan, place it over medium heat, grease it with oil and when hot, add sausage and cook for 3 minutes per side until sauté.
3. Place eggs and egg whites in a bowl, whisk until blended, then add sausage, spinach, and potatoes and mix well until combined.
4. Take a 9 by 13 inches casserole dish or six heatproof meal prep glass containers, spoon in sausage mixture, and bake the casserole for 45 minutes until thoroughly cooked.
5. For meal prepping, let casserole or containers cool completely, then cover the casserole well with aluminum foil or close the containers with lid and store in the refrigerator for up to five days or freeze for three months.
6. Reheat casserole in the microwave until hot and serve.

Nutrition Value:

- Calories: 258.4 Cal
- Fat: 12.8 g
- Carbs: 13 g
- Protein: 22.8 g
- Fiber: 5 g

Omelet Muffins

Preparation time: 10 minutes
Cooking time: 40 minutes
Servings: 6

Ingredients:

- 4 scallions, sliced
- 2 cups chopped broccoli
- 3 slices of bacon, chopped
- ½ teaspoon ground black pepper
- ½ teaspoon salt
- 8 eggs
- ½ cup milk
- 1 cup shredded cheddar cheese

Method:

1. Switch on the oven, then set it to 325 degrees F and let it preheat.
2. Meanwhile, take a skillet pan, place it over medium heat and when hot, add bacon and cook for 5 minutes until cooked and crispy.
3. Transfer cooked bacon to a plate lined with paper towels and set aside until required.
4. Add scallion and broccoli into the pan, stir well and cook for 5 minutes until softened, set aside and let cool for 5 minutes.
5. In the meantime, place cheese in a bowl, add eggs, pour in milk, season with black pepper and salt, and whisk until combined.
6. Then add bacon and broccoli and stir until well mixed.
7. Take a twelve cups muffin pan, grease its cups with oil, then fill the cups evenly with broccoli mixture and bake for 30 minutes until firm.
8. When done, take out muffins from the pan and let them cool on a wire rack.
9. For meal prep, wrap each muffin with aluminum foil and refrigerate for up to five days or freeze for up to one month.
10. When ready to eat, reheat the muffin in the microwave until hot and serve.

Nutrition Value:

- Calories: 211 Cal
- Fat: 14 g
- Carbs: 5 g
- Protein: 16 g
- Fiber: 1 g

Parsnip Hash Browns

Preparation time: 10 minutes
Cooking time: 10 minutes
Servings: 6

Ingredients:

- 16 ounces waxy potato
- 12 ounces parsnip
- 1 small white onion, halved and sliced
- ½ tablespoon minced garlic
- 1 egg, beaten
- 4 tablespoons olive oil

Method:

1. Peel the potatoes and parsnip, grate them by using a food processor, then wrap potatoes and parsnip in a kitchen cloth and squeeze out moisture as much as possible.
2. Place squeeze potatoes and parsnip in a bowl, add egg, garlic, and onion and whisk until well combined.
3. Shape the mixture into six flat cakes, then place them on a cookie sheet lined with parchment paper and freeze until hard.
4. For meal prep, transfer frozen the hash browns in a plastic bag and freeze in the freezer for up to three months.
5. When ready to eat, place a skillet over medium heat, add oil and hash brown and cook for 15 minutes until hot and nicely browned on both sides, flipping every 5 minutes.
6. Serve hash browns with cherry tomatoes and poached eggs.

Nutrition Value:

- Calories: 179 Cal
- Fat: 9 g
- Carbs: 21 g
- Protein: 4 g
- Fiber: 4 g

Chapter 5: Poultry

Buffalo Chicken Casserole

Preparation time: 10 minutes
Cooking time: 55 minutes
Servings: 4

Ingredients:

- 1/2 cup diced carrots
- 15 ounces cauliflower florets, riced
- 1 small white onion, peeled, diced
- ½ teaspoon minced garlic
- 1 pound chicken breast, skinless, cooked, shredded
- 1/4 teaspoon ground black pepper
- 2 tablespoons olive oil
- 1/2 cup egg whites
- 3/4 cup buffalo sauce

Method:

1. Switch on the oven, then set it to 400 degrees F and let it preheat.
2. Take a skillet pan, place it over medium heat, add oil and when hot, add onion, celery, and carrots and cook for 5 minutes or until softened.
3. Then transfer vegetables to a bowl, add remaining ingredients and mix well until combined.
4. Take a baking pan or casserole dish, line it with parchment sheet, spoon in the prepared mixture, then cover with aluminum foil and bake for 25 minutes.
5. Uncover the pan and continue baking for 25 minutes until casserole has set and the top is nicely golden brown.
6. When the casserole has cooked, remove it from the oven and let it cool completely.
7. Then divide the casserole into four pieces and place each casserole piece in a heatproof glass meal prep container.
8. Cover meal prep containers with lid and freeze for up to two months.
9. When ready to eat, reheat the casserole in the microwave until hot, cover the top if it gets too brown, and then serve with a green salad.

Nutrition Value:

- Calories: 256 Cal
- Fat: 13 g
- Carbs: 13 g
- Protein: 24 g
- Fiber: 4 g

Chicken Mason Jar Salad

Preparation time: 10 minutes
Cooking time: 0 minute
Servings: 4

Ingredients:

For the Salad:

- 2 tablespoons sliced green onions
- 2 cups sliced napa cabbage
- 1 cup grated carrots
- 1 1/3 cup snap peas, halved
- 2 cups shredded rotisserie chicken
- 1 red pepper, julienned
- 1 1/3 cups cucumber, sliced
- 2 cups baby spinach, sliced
- 1 cup cashews, unsalted

For the Sesame Dressing:

- 1 tablespoon minced ginger
- 2 tablespoons diced cilantro
- 3 tablespoons soy sauce
- 1 tablespoon honey
- 1 tablespoon olive oil
- ½ teaspoon minced garlic
- 2 tablespoons apple cider vinegar
- 2 1/2 tablespoons sesame oil
- 1 teaspoon sriracha sauce
- 1 teaspoon sesame seeds

Method:

1. Prepare the dressing and for this, place all its ingredients in a bowl and whisk until combined.
2. Place cabbage in a bowl, add spinach and toss until combined.
3. Assemble the salad jar and for this, take four 64-ounce mason salad jar, and working on one mason jar at a time, spoon 3 tablespoons of prepared salad dressing into a salad jar, add 1/3 cup snap peas and top with ¼ cup shredded carrots.
4. Add 1/3 cup cucumber, top with 1 cup of cabbage mixture, ½ cup chicken, then add ¼ cup cashews and sprinkle with green onions.
5. Prepare remaining salad jars in the same manner, cover with the lid, and store in the freezer for up to four days.
6. Serve straight away.

Nutrition Value:

- Calories: 524 Cal
- Fat: 33 g
- Carbs: 39 g
- Protein: 28 g
- Fiber: 5 g

Chicken Meatballs

Preparation time: 15 minutes
Cooking time: 40 minutes
Servings: 4

Ingredients:

For the veggie:

- 1 pound fingerling potatoes, quartered
- ½ teaspoon salt
- 2 tablespoons avocado oil
- 1 white onion, peeled, cut into large chunks
- ½ teaspoon cumin
- 1 ½ tablespoon minced garlic

For the meatballs:

- 1 pound ground chicken
- 1 tablespoon coconut flour
- ½ teaspoon salt
- 1 teaspoon ground turmeric
- 2 tablespoons parsley
- 1 teaspoon ground cumin
- 2 tablespoons cilantro
- 1/2 teaspoon garlic powder
- ½ teaspoon ground black pepper
- 1 teaspoon Dijon mustard
- 1 egg

For the Green Tahini Sauce:

- 2 tablespoons chopped parsley
- ¼ cup tahini
- 2 tablespoons chopped cilantro
- 2 tablespoons lemon juice
- ¼ teaspoon salt
- 2 tablespoons warm water

Method:

1. Switch on the oven, then set it to 400 degrees F and let preheat.
2. Take a baking sheet, line it with parchment sheet, add potatoes on it along with onion and garlic.
3. Season with salt and cumin, drizzle with oil, and then toss with hands until potatoes are well coated.
4. Spread the potatoes evenly in the baking sheet and bake for 20 minutes.
5. Meanwhile, prepare the meatballs and for this, place all its ingredients in a bowl, stir well until combined and shape the mixture into twelve meatballs.
6. After 20 minutes of baking time, take out the baking sheet, stir the potatoes, then move them to one side of the sheet, place meatballs in the vacant space of the

baking sheet and continue baking for 20 to 23 minutes until thoroughly cooked and golden brown.

7. In the meantime, prepare the tahini sauce, and for this, place all its ingredients in a blender or food processor and pulse for 30 seconds until smooth; blend in more water if the sauce is too thick.

8. For meal prep, let potatoes and meatballs cool completely.

9. Then evenly place spinach in the bottom of four heatproof meal prep containers, then portion the meatballs on one side and potatoes to another side.

10. Cover the containers with lid and store in the refrigerator for up to a week.

11. When ready to eat, reheat potatoes and meatballs in the microwave and then serve with tahini sauce.

Nutrition Value:

- Calories: 448.7 Cal
- Fat: 24.7 g
- Carbs: 29.5 g

- Protein: 30.2 g
- Fiber: 5.8 g

Honey Sesame Chicken

Preparation time: 10 minutes
Cooking time: 15 minutes
Servings: 4

Ingredients:

For the Honey Sesame Sauce:

- 1/4 cup honey
- 1/2 teaspoon red pepper flakes
- 1/4 cup chicken stock
- 1 tablespoon sesame oil
- 1/4 cup soy sauce
- 1 teaspoon cornstarch

For Meal Prepping:

- 3 cups broccoli florets, chopped
- 2 large chicken breasts, cut into small pieces
- 3/4 cup rice, cooked
- ½ teaspoon ground black pepper
- 3 cups snap peas, chopped
- 2/3 teaspoon salt
- 1 tablespoon olive oil
- 1 teaspoon sesame seeds

Method:

1. Prepare the sauce and for this, place all its ingredients in a bowl and whisk until combined, set aside until required.
2. Take a large skillet pan, place it over medium heat, add oil and when hot, add peas and broccoli, and cook for 5 minutes until vegetables are tender and bright green.
3. In the meantime, evenly divide the cooked rice between four heatproof meal prep containers.
4. Add cooked peas and broccoli evenly into the meal prep container and return pan over the heat.
5. Add chicken pieces, season with red pepper, black pepper, and salt and cook for 7 minutes until thoroughly cooked.
6. Pour in the prepared sauce, stir until mixed and simmer for 2 minutes until the sauce has thickened slightly.
7. Evenly add chicken into meal prep containers, then drizzle chicken with sauce, and garnish with sesame seeds.
8. Cover the containers with a lid and refrigerate for up to a week.
9. When ready to eat, reheat the container into the microwave until hot and then serve.

Nutrition Value:

- Calories: 445 Cal
- Fat: 11 g
- Carbs: 56 g

- Protein: 33 g
- Fiber: 3 g

Lemon Herb Chicken with Vegetables

Preparation time: 10 minutes
Cooking time: 20 minutes
Servings: 4

Ingredients:

For the Chicken:

- 2 chicken breasts, skinless, pounded
- 1 teaspoon honey
- 1 teaspoon lemon zest
- 3 tablespoons olive oil
- 4 tablespoons lemon juice

For the Seasonings:

- 1/2 teaspoon smoked paprika
- 1/4 teaspoon ground black pepper
- 1/2 teaspoon dried thyme
- 2 teaspoons sea salt
- 1/2 teaspoon dried oregano
- 1/2 teaspoon garlic powder

For the Vegetables:

- 1/2 cup purple baby potatoes, halved
- 1/2 cup cherry tomatoes, halved
- 1/2 red bell pepper, 1 inch cubed
- 1/3 cup snap peas
- 1/3 cup chopped carrots
- 1/3 cup broccoli florets
- ½ of medium orange bell pepper, 1 inch cubed
- 1/2 cup baby potatoes, halved
- 1/3 of medium yellow bell pepper, 1 inch cubed
- 1/3 cup chopped zucchini
- 1/2 cup radishes

For Serving:

- Cooked quinoa as needed

Method:

1. Switch on the oven, then set it to 400 degrees F, and let preheat.
2. Prepare the marinade and for this, place all the seasonings in a bowl, add honey, oil, lemon juice, and zest and whisk until combined.
3. Pour half of the marinade in a large plastic bag, add chicken, seal the bag, then turn it upside down to coat chicken with marinade and then rub it into the meat.
4. Add all the vegetables into the remaining marinade, one at a time, and toss until well coated.

5. Take a large baking sheet, line it with aluminum foil, arrange vegetables in it in separate rows, then add chicken and bake for 8 minutes.
6. Then flip the chicken, toss the vegetables, and continue baking for 12 minutes until the chicken has thoroughly cooked.
7. Let the vegetables and chicken cool, portion them into four heatproof glass meal prep containers, then evenly add quinoa.
8. Cover the containers with a lid and refrigerate for up to five days or freeze for up to one month.
9. When ready to eat, reheat the container in the microwave until hot and then serve.

Nutrition Value:

- Calories: 231 Cal
- Fat: 12 g
- Carbs: 16 g
- Protein: 14 g
- Fiber: 3 g

Caprese Chicken Salad

Preparation time: 20 minutes
Cooking time: 28 minutes
Servings: 4

Ingredients:

- 1 cup baby bocconcini
- 14 ounces chicken breasts
- 2 cups cooked quinoa
- 3 cups cherry tomatoes, halved
- 1 bunch of basil leaves

- 1 teaspoon ground black pepper
- 1 teaspoon salt
- 1 tablespoon olive oil
- 1 tablespoon apple cider vinegar

For the Balsamic Vinaigrette:

- 1 tablespoon maple syrup
- ¼ teaspoon ground black pepper
- ¼ teaspoon salt

- 1/4 teaspoon Dijon mustard
- 3 tablespoons apple cider vinegar
- 3 tablespoons olive oil

Method:

1. Switch on the oven, then set it to 425 degrees F, and let preheat.
2. Meanwhile, place chicken in a shallow dish, drizzle with vinegar and 1 tablespoon oil, season with salt and black pepper, toss until well coated and bake for 25 to 28 minutes until thoroughly cooked.
3. Then let the chicken cool for 10 minutes and cut into cubes.
4. Prepare the vinaigrette and for this, place all its ingredients in a bowl and whisk until blended.
5. For meal prepping, divide chicken cubes evenly between heatproof glass meal prep containers, add ½ cup quinoa, ¾ cup tomato halves, ¼ cup bocconcini, and some basil leaves.
6. Drizzle with prepared vinaigrette, cover the containers with a lid and refrigerate for up to five days or freeze for up to two months.
7. When ready to eat, reheat the container in the microwave until hot and then serve.

Nutrition Value:

- Calories: 464 Cal
- Fat: 23 g
- Carbs: 31 g

- Protein: 31 g
- Fiber: 3 g

Vietnamese Chicken

Preparation time: 15 minutes
Cooking time: 26 minutes
Servings: 4

Ingredients:

- 1 1/4 cups brown rice, uncooked
- 2 large carrots, peeled, cut into thin strips
- 2 large hands full of sugar snap peas, ends trimmed, halved vertically
- 2 pounds chicken thighs, boneless
- 4 tablespoons honey
- 1 tablespoon fish sauce
- 4 tablespoons apple cider vinegar
- 1 tablespoon soy sauce
- 2 tablespoons olive oil
- 2 cups chicken broth
- 4 tablespoons sesame seeds

For the marinade:

- 2 tablespoons honey
- 1 tablespoon fish sauce
- 1 tablespoon soy sauce

Method:

1. Prepare the marinade and for this, place all its ingredients in a large bowl and whisk until combined.
2. Cut chicken thighs into cubes, add them to the marinade, toss until well coated, and let it rest for 10 minutes.
3. Meanwhile, prepare the rice and for this, place a saucepan over medium heat, pour in chicken broth and bring it to boil.
4. Then add rice, stir well and cook for 3 to 5 minutes until rice is tender, fluff the rice with fork and set aside.
5. Cook the vegetables and for this, take a large pan over medium heat, add 1 tablespoon oil and when hot, add carrot and snap peas and sauté for 3 to 4 minutes until tender-crisp, set aside until required.
6. Then add remaining oil in the pan, add chicken pieces in a single layer and cook for 2 minutes per side.
7. Transfer the chicken pieces to a plate and cook the remaining chicken cubes in the same manner.
8. Prepare the sauce and for this, add vinegar, soy sauce, fish sauce, and honey into the pan, stir well, then bring it to boil and cook for 2 to 3 minutes until the sauce has thickened slightly.

9. Then return the chicken into the pan, stir until chicken is coated with sauce and cook for 2 minutes, remove the pan from heat.
10. For meal prep, evenly divide brown rice, vegetables, and brown rice evenly in four heatproof meal prep containers, then sprinkle sesame seeds over the chicken and let it cool completely.
11. Cover the containers with a lid and refrigerate for up to five days or freeze for up to one month.
12. When ready to eat, reheat the container in the microwave until hot and then serve.

Nutrition Value:

- Calories: 654 Cal
- Fat: 14 g
- Carbs: 78 g
- Protein: 51 g
- Fiber: 2 g

Cashew Chicken

Preparation time: 15 minutes
Cooking time: 25 minutes
Servings: 4

Ingredients:

For the Chicken and Vegetables:

- 2 medium chicken breasts
- 1 red bell pepper, cored, cut into chunks
- 1 ½ cups broccoli florets
- ½ green bell pepper, cored, cut into chunks
- 1 teaspoon ground black pepper
- 1 ½ teaspoon salt
- 2/3 cup roasted cashews, unsalted

For the Sauce:

- 2 tablespoons arrowroot starch
- 1 tablespoon minced garlic
- 6 tablespoons soy sauce
- ½ teaspoon minced ginger
- ¾ tablespoon apple cider vinegar
- 2 tablespoons honey
- 1 teaspoon toasted sesame oil
- ½ cup water and more as needed

For Serving:

- 2 cups cooked brown rice
- 2 tablespoons sesame seeds

Method:

1. Switch on the oven, then set it to 400 degrees F, and let it preheat.
2. Prepare the sauce and for this, place all its ingredients in a saucepan, whisk well until combined, then bring it to simmer over medium heat and cook for 3 minutes until thickened, set aside until required.
3. Prepare the chicken and vegetables and for this, cut the chicken into 1-inch cubes, and place them in a shallow dish.
4. Season the chicken with ½ teaspoon black pepper and ¾ teaspoon salt, drizzle with half of the prepared sauce, and toss until well coated on all sides.
5. Take a large sheet pan, line it with aluminum foil, spray with oil, then spread chicken cubes on it and cook for 8 minutes.
6. Then add cashew, bell peppers, and broccoli florets around the chicken in a single layer, season with remaining salt and black pepper, drizzle with half of the remaining sauce and toss until well coated.

7. Continue baking for 12 minutes until the chicken has thoroughly cooked, then remove the baking sheet from the oven, drizzle with remaining sauce and let cool completely.
8. Evenly divide cashew chicken and vegetables into four heatproof meal prep containers, add cooked brown rice to one side of the container and then sprinkle sesame seeds over chicken.
9. Cover the containers with a lid and refrigerate for up to five days or freeze for up to one month.
10. When ready to eat, reheat the container in the microwave until hot and then serve.

Nutrition Value:

- Calories: 251 Cal
- Fat: 11 g
- Carbs: 27 g
- Protein: 12 g
- Fiber: 2 g

Cilantro Lime Chicken with Cauliflower Rice

Preparation time: 25 minutes
Cooking time: 25 minutes
Servings: 4

Ingredients:

For the Chicken:

- 1 pound chicken breast
- 1/3 cup chopped fresh cilantro
- ¾ teaspoon ground black pepper
- 2 teaspoons minced garlic
- 1 ½ teaspoon salt
- 1/2 teaspoon honey
- 1/4 cup lime juice
- 2 tablespoons olive oil

For the Cauliflower Rice:

- 3 cups cauliflower rice
- 1/2 cup cooked black beans
- 2 teaspoons garlic powder
- 1/4 cup chopped red onion
- 1 teaspoon ground cumin
- 1/8 sea salt
- 2 tablespoons olive oil

For Serving:

- 1 cup cherry tomatoes, halved
- 1 medium avocado, peeled, pitted, chopped

Method:

1. Prepare the chicken for this, take a skillet pan, place it over medium heat, add oil and when hot, add chicken and cook for 5 to 8 minutes per side until nicely browned.
2. Transfer chicken to a cutting board, let it cool for 15 minutes and then cut it into slices.
3. Place remaining ingredients For the chicken in a bowl, whisk well until mixed, add chicken slices, then toss until well coated and refrigerate until required.
4. Prepare the cauliflower rice and for this, return the skillet pan over medium heat, add oil and when hot, add cauliflower rice, season with garlic powder, cumin, and salt, stir well and cook for 5 minutes.
5. Add beans, continue cooking for 2 minutes until heated, then add red onion, stir well and cook for 2 minutes, let cool completely.
6. Evenly divide chicken and cauliflower into four heatproof meal prep containers and then add tomatoes and avocado.

7. Cover the containers with a lid and refrigerate for up to five days.
8. When ready to eat, reheat the chicken and cauliflower rice in the microwave until hot and then serve.

Nutrition Value:

- Calories: 378 Cal
- Fat: 21 g
- Carbs: 16 g
- Protein: 32 g
- Fiber: 7 g

Turkey Taco

Preparation time: 15 minutes
Cooking time: 45 minutes
Servings: 4

Ingredients:

For the Rice:

- 1/8 teaspoon salt
- 3/4 cup brown rice, uncooked
- 1 lime, zested
- 1 ½ cups water

For Turkey:

- 2 tablespoons taco seasoning
- 3/4 pound ground turkey

For the Salsa:

- 1/4 cup minced red onion
- 2 cups cherry tomatoes, quartered
- 1/8 teaspoon salt
- 1 jalapeno pepper, minced
- 2 tablespoons lime juice

For Serving:

- 1/4 cup shredded cheese cheddar or mozzarella

Method:

1. Prepare the rice and for this, take a saucepan, place it over medium heat, add rice and water, and bring it to boil.
2. Then reduce heat to medium-low level, add salt and lime zest, cover the pan and cook for 30 to 45 minutes until rice has absorbed water and cooked through.
3. Meanwhile, cook the turkey and for this, take a skillet pan, place it over medium heat and when hot, add turkey, break it up, season with taco seasoning and cook for 10 minutes until nicely browned and thoroughly cooked.
4. While turkey is cooking, prepare the salsa and for this, place all its ingredients in a bowl, toss until well mixed and refrigerate until required.
5. When the rice has cooked, remove the pan from heat, fluff them with a fork and cool for 15 minutes.
6. Evenly divide rice into four heatproof meal prep containers, then add ½ cup turkey taco and ½ cup salsa and sprinkle cheese on top of the turkey.
7. Cover the containers with a lid and refrigerate for up to five days.

8. When ready to eat, reheat the rice and turkey taco in the microwave until hot and then serve.

Nutrition Value:

- Calories: 387 Cal
- Fat: 10 g
- Carbs: 42 g

- Protein: 23 g
- Fiber: 5 g

Chapter 6: Snacks and Siders

Stuffed Portobello Mushrooms

Preparation time: 10 minutes
Cooking time: 10 minutes
Servings: 2

Ingredients:

- 6 large portobello mushrooms
- 6 slices of a large tomato
- 1/8 teaspoon ground black pepper
- ½ teaspoon minced garlic
- 2 tablespoons olive oil
- 2 tablespoons minced parsley
- 3/4 cup fresh basil leaves
- 3/4 cup ricotta cheese
- 3 tablespoons slivered almonds
- 1/2 cup shredded mozzarella cheese
- 3/4 cup grated Parmesan cheese, divided
- 3 teaspoons water

Method:

1. Place ¼ cup of parmesan cheese in a bowl, add ricotta and mozzarella cheese along with black pepper and parsley and stir until mixed.
2. Remove stem from each mushroom, remove the gills by scrapping with a spoon, then stuff with cheese mixture and top each stuffed mushroom with a tomato slice.
3. Take a griddle pan, place it over medium heat, grease the pan with oil, place stuffed mushrooms on it, and cook for 10 minutes until tender.
4. Meanwhile, place basil leaves in a food processor, add garlic and almond, and pulse for 1 minute until chopped.
5. Blend in remaining cheese and then blend in oil and water in a steady stream until mixture reach to desired consistency.
6. Let mushrooms cool completely, then portion between two heatproof glass meal prep containers, cover the containers with lid, and then freeze for up to one month.
7. When ready to eat, reheat the mushrooms until hot, then top with cheese mixture and serve.

Nutrition Value:

- Calories: 201 Cal
- Fat: 13 g
- Carbs: 9 g
- Protein: 12 g
- Fiber: 2 g

Jalapeno Sliders

Preparation time: 10 minutes
Cooking time: 20 minutes
Servings: 2

Ingredients:

- 1 pound ground beef
- 1 large sweet potato
- 1 small jalapeno, diced
- 1/2 teaspoon garlic powder
- 2/3 teaspoon ground black pepper
- 1/2 teaspoon cumin
- 1 teaspoon salt
- 1 tablespoon olive oil

Method:

1. Switch on the oven, then set it to 425 degrees F, and let it preheat.
2. Rinse the sweet potatoes, cut into horizontally into eight thick slices and then place them on a baking sheet lined with aluminum foil.
3. Drizzle oil over sweet potato slices, season with salt and black pepper, and then bake for 20 minutes until cooked.
4. Meanwhile, place beef in a bowl, add garlic powder, cumin, and jalapeno, mix well and shape the mixture into four patties.
5. Take a grill pan, place it over medium heat, grease with oil and when hot, add patties on it and cook for 4 minutes per side until browned and thoroughly cooked.
6. When patties and sweet potatoes have cooked, let them cool completely.
7. For meal prep, take two heatproof glass meal prep containers, place two sweet potato slices into each container, then top with a patty and cover patty with a sweet potato slice.
8. Shut the containers with lid and refrigerate for up to five days.
9. When ready to eat, reheat the containers in the microwave until hot and serve.

Nutrition Value:

- Calories: 483 Cal
- Fat: 23 g
- Carbs: 21 g
- Protein: 48 g
- Fiber: 9 g

Peanut Butter Energy Bites

Preparation time: 40 minutes
Cooking time: 0 minute
Servings: 18

Ingredients:

- 2 tablespoons ground flax
- 1 1/2 cups rolled oats
- 1/4 cup chia seeds
- 2 tablespoons cocoa powder, unsweetened
- 1/2 cup protein powder
- 2 tablespoons agave syrup
- 1/2 cup peanut butter
- 1 cup water

Method:

1. Place chia seeds in a bowl, pour in water, stir in protein powder, stir until mixed and refrigerate for 5 minutes.
2. Then place remaining ingredients in another bowl, add chia seeds mixture, stir until well combined and then with a wet hand, shape the mixture into 1-inch balls, about eighteen.
3. Place balls on a sheet pan lined with parchment paper and freeze for 30 minutes until firm.
4. Store the energy balls in the refrigerator for up to one week, or transfer them into a freezer-proof bag and freeze for up to one month.

Nutrition Value:

- Calories: 117 Cal
- Fat: 5 g
- Carbs: 10 g
- Protein: 8 g
- Fiber: 3 g

Thai Turkey Lettuce Wraps

Preparation time: 10 minutes
Cooking time: 10 minutes
Servings: 6

Ingredients:

For the Sauce:

- 3 tablespoons soy sauce
- 1 tablespoon lime juice
- 2 tablespoons rice vinegar
- 1/4 cup peanut butter
- 1 teaspoon sesame oil
- 2 tablespoons water

For the Filling:

- 1 pound ground turkey
- 1 medium white onion, peeled, chopped
- 1 cup shredded carrots
- 1 tablespoon minced garlic
- 1 tablespoon Thai red curry paste
- 1 tablespoon olive oil

For Serving:

- Green onions as needed to garnish
- 7 ounces Romaine lettuce leaf
- Peanuts as needed to garnish

Method:

1. Prepare the sauce and for this, place all the ingredients For the sauce in a bowl, whisk well until combined, and set aside until required.
2. Prepare the filling and for this, take a skillet pan, place it over medium heat, add oil and when hot, add garlic, onion and curry paste, stir well and cook for 3 minutes until heated.
3. Then add turkey, break it up, stir well and continue cooking for 7 minutes until turkey is no longer pink and thoroughly cooked.
4. Add carrots and peanut sauce, stir until mixed, and then remove the pan from heat.
5. For meal prep, let the turkey mixture cool completely and then evenly portion between six heatproof glass meal prep containers.
6. Cover the containers with a lid, store them in the refrigerator for up to four days or freeze for up to one month.
7. When ready to eat, thaw the frozen turkey mixture and then reheat in the microwave oven until hot.

8. Stuff the turkey mixture in lettuce leaves, top with green onions and peanuts, and serve.

Nutrition Value:

- Calories: 264 Cal
- Fat: 15 g
- Carbs: 13 g

- Protein: 20 g
- Fiber: 4 g

Chipotle Honey Chicken Taco Salad

Preparation time: 10 minutes
Cooking time: 4 hours
Servings: 4

Ingredients:

For the Chicken:

- 2 chicken breasts
- ½ teaspoon minced garlic
- 1/4 teaspoon salt
- 1/4 cup honey
- 1 tablespoon lime juice
- 2 tablespoons adobo sauce
- 1/4 cup chicken stock

For the Salad:

- 1 medium green bell pepper, sliced
- 2 medium carrots, peeled, shredded
- 3 cups shredded cabbage

For Serving:

- Tortilla chips as needed

Method:

1. Prepare the chicken and for this, place chicken in a slow cooker, add remaining ingredients and toss until well coated.
2. Switch on the slow cooker, shut it with lid and cook for 4 hours at low heat setting or for 3 hours at high heat setting until chicken is tender, don't overcook.
3. Let the chicken cool completely, then evenly divide it between four glass meal prep containers and drizzle with sauce.
4. Cover the containers with the lid, store them in the refrigerator for up to four days or freeze for up to one month.
5. When ready to eat, thaw the frozen chicken and then reheat in the microwave oven until hot.
6. Let chicken cool slightly, then add the ingredients For the salad and toss until mixed.
7. Top the chicken salad with tortilla chips and serve.

Nutrition Value:

- Calories: 253 Cal
- Fat: 5 g
- Carbs: 27 g
- Protein: 24 g
- Fiber: 4 g

Sweet Potato, Lentil, and Kale Salad

Preparation time: 10 minutes
Cooking time: 35 minutes
Servings: 4

Ingredients:

For the Salad:

- 3/4 cup brown lentils, uncooked
- 4 cups cubed sweet potato, peeled
- 2 teaspoons olive oil
- 4 cups chopped kale
- 1 large red bell pepper, cored, diced
- 1/4 cup diced red onion
- 3 teaspoons salt
- 1 teaspoon ground black pepper
- ¼ cup roasted pumpkin seeds
- 1 ½ cup water

For the Tahini Dressing:

- 1/3 cup tahini
- ½ tablespoon minced garlic
- 1/4 teaspoon salt
- 1/2 teaspoon curry powder
- 2 tablespoons lemon juice
- 7 tablespoons water

Method:

1. Switch on the oven, then set it to 375 degrees F and let preheat.
2. Take a large sheet pan, add sweet potato cubes on it, drizzle with oil, then sprinkle with 1 ½ teaspoon salt and black pepper, toss until mixed and bake for 35 minutes until tender, stirring halfway through.
3. Meanwhile, prepare the lentils and for this, take a medium saucepan, place it over medium heat, pour in water, add lentils and ½ teaspoon salt, bring it to simmer, and then cook for 20 minutes until lentils are tender, let cool completely.
4. Prepare the dressing and for this, place all its ingredients in a bowl and whisk until combined, set aside until required.
5. Prepare kale and for this, place kale in a bowl, season with remaining salt, drizzle with lemon juice, then massage the kale leaves for 30 seconds until slightly softened and set aside.
6. Assemble the salad and for this, take four mason jars, spoon 2 tablespoons of prepared dressing in the bottom of each jar, then add ½ cup of cooked lentils, top with ½ cup baked sweet potato and ¼ of diced red peppers, and then add 1 tablespoon onion and 1 cup kale leaves.
7. Prepare three more mason salad jars in the same manner, then tighten with lid and refrigerate for four days.

8. When ready to eat, top the salad with a tablespoon of pumpkin seeds and serve.

Nutrition Value:

- Calories: 400 Cal
- Fat: 18 g
- Carbs: 43 g
- Protein: 13 g
- Fiber: 15 g

Peanut-Lime Chicken Bowl

Preparation time: 15 minutes
Cooking time: 30 minutes
Servings: 4

Ingredients:

For the Rice:

- 3/4 cup brown rice, uncooked
- 3/4 cup chicken stock
- 3/4 cup water
- 1/4 teaspoon salt
- 1 tablespoon lime zest

For the Chicken:

- 16 ounces chicken breasts
- 1 tablespoon olive oil
- 1 tablespoon soy sauce

For the Vegetables:

- 2 cups diced carrots
- 2 cups broccoli florets
- 1 tablespoon olive oil

For the Peanut Lime Sauce:

- 1/4 cup peanut butter
- 1 1/2 tablespoons apple cider vinegar
- 1/2 tablespoon brown sugar
- 1/2 teaspoon sesame oil
- 1/2 tablespoon lime juice
- 2 tablespoons of water or more as needed to thin it out

For Serving

- 1/4 cup peanuts

Method:

1. Switch on the oven, then set it to 425 degrees F, and let preheat.
2. Cook the rice and for this, place a saucepan over medium-high heat, add all the ingredients for rice, stir well and bring it to boil.
3. Then reduce heat to medium-low level and simmer rice for 20 minutes or more until the rice has absorbed all the liquid and tender, fluff the cooked rice with a fork, and set aside.

4. Prepare the chicken and for this, place chicken in a small baking pan, drizzle with oil and soy sauce, toss until well coated on both sides, and then bake for 20 minutes until cooked through, flipping the chicken halfway.
5. Meanwhile, take a large baking sheet, place carrot and broccoli florets on it, drizzle with oil, toss until well coated and bake the vegetables with chicken for 20 minutes until roasted, stirring halfway through.
6. Prepare the sauce and for this, place peanut butter in a heatproof bowl, microwave for 30 seconds, then stir until smooth, add remaining ingredients For the sauce and whisk until well combined, whisk in 2 tablespoons water if the sauce is too thick.
7. For meal prep, cool the chicken and vegetables, then divide them evenly between for glass meal prep containers, add boiled rice and then drizzle 2 tablespoons of prepared sauce over chicken in each container.
8. Cover the containers with the lid, store them in the refrigerator for up to five days or freeze for up to one month.
9. When ready to eat, thaw the frozen chicken and vegetables, and then reheat in the microwave oven until hot.
10. Sprinkle peanuts over chicken and serve.

Nutrition Value:

- Calories: 495 Cal
- Fat: 19 g
- Carbs: 49 g
- Protein: 36 g
- Fiber: 6 g

Mediterranean Chickpea Salad

Preparation time: 10 minutes
Cooking time: 0 minute
Servings: 6

Ingredients:

For the Chickpea Salad:

- 1 cup cubed cucumber
- 1 1/2 cups chickpeas, cooked
- 1/2 cup chopped parsley leaves
- 1/2 of large red onion, peeled, chopped
- 1 cup cubed cherry tomatoes
- 1/4 cup feta cheese, crumbled

For the Vinaigrette

- 1/4 teaspoon ground black pepper
- 1/2 teaspoon sea salt
- 1 teaspoon Dijon mustard
- 2 teaspoons lemon juice
- 1/4 cup olive oil
- 1 tablespoon apple cider vinegar

Method:

1. Place all the ingredients For the salad in a bowl and toss until just mixed.
2. Prepare the vinaigrette and for this, place all its ingredients in another bowl and whisk until combined.
3. Drizzle with vinaigrette over chickpea salad, toss until well mixed and then portion it between three meal prep containers.
4. Tighten the containers with lid and store in the refrigerator for up to four days.
5. Serve when ready to eat.

Nutrition Value:

- Calories: 339.8 Cal
- Fat: 13.7 g
- Carbs: 44.4 g
- Protein: 12.1 g
- Fiber: 8.8 g

Almond Butter Turkey Meatballs

Preparation time: 10 minutes
Cooking time: 12 minutes
Servings: 4

Ingredients:

For the Meatballs:

- 1 pound ground turkey breast
- 1 teaspoon garlic powder
- 1 teaspoon onion powder
- ½ teaspoon ground ginger

For Peanut Butter Sauce:

- 2 tablespoons red curry paste
- 1 tablespoon coconut sugar
- 1/2 cup almond butter
- 1 tablespoon soy sauce
- 1 tablespoon apple cider vinegar
- 4 tablespoons lime juice
- 3/4 cup coconut milk

Method:

1. Switch on the oven, then set it to 425 degrees F, and let it preheat.
2. Prepare the sauce and for this, place all its ingredients in a bowl and whisk until combined.
3. Place all the ingredients for meatballs in another bowl, mix well and then shape the mixture into fourteen meatballs.
4. Take a skillet pan, grease it with oil, spread ¼ cup of the sauce and then place meatballs in it.
5. Top the meatballs with remaining sauce and bake for 12 minutes until meatballs have thoroughly cooked.
6. Let meatballs cool completely, then pour the meatballs and sauce evenly between four heatproof glass meal prep containers and tighten with lid.
7. Store the containers in the refrigerator for up to four days or freeze for up to one month.
8. When ready to eat, thaw the meatballs, then reheat in the microwave until hot and serve.

Nutrition Value:

- Calories: 355 Cal
- Fat: 19 g
- Carbs: 10 g
- Protein: 36 g
- Fiber: 3 g

Chipotle Shredded Chicken

Preparation time: 10 minutes
Cooking time: 30 minutes
Servings: 4

Ingredients:

- 1 pound chicken breasts
- 3 chipotle peppers in adobo sauce, minced
- 1 ½ teaspoon minced garlic
- 1 teaspoon adobo sauce
- 1/2 cup chopped fresh cilantro,
- 2 teaspoons yellow mustard
- 1 tablespoon olive oil
- 2 cups chicken broth
- 1 cup orange juice, unsweetened

Method:

1. Take a large pot, place it over medium heat, add oil and when hot, add garlic and chipotle pepper and cook for 2 minutes until sauté, stirring continuously.
2. Switch heat to the high level, add cilantro, pour in chicken broth and orange juice, stir well and bring the mixture to boil.
3. Then add chicken, switch heat to medium-low level and simmer for 15 to 20 minutes until the chicken has thoroughly cooked.
4. When done, transfer chicken to a cutting board, let it rest for 5 minutes, and then shred it with two forks.
5. In the meantime, whisk mustard into the sauce and continue cooking the sauce over low heat until reduced by half.
6. Return the shredded chicken into the pot, toss until well coated in sauce, and then let cool.
7. For meal prep, divide chicken evenly between four glass meal prep containers, tighten them with lid and refrigerate for up to three days or freeze for up to one month.
8. When ready to eat, thaw the chicken, then reheat in the microwave until hot and serve.

Nutrition Value:

- Calories: 148 Cal
- Fat: 4.5 g
- Carbs: 5.4 g
- Protein: 18.3 g
- Fiber: 0.2 g

Chapter 7: Beef and Pork

Honey-Chipotle Meatball

Preparation time: 15 minutes
Cooking time: 30 minutes
Servings: 4

Ingredients:

For the Meatballs:

- 1 pound ground beef
- 1/2 teaspoon salt
- 1 teaspoon Worcestershire sauce
- 1 egg
- 1/2 cup breadcrumbs

For Chipotle Glaze

- 1 chipotle pepper
- 1/2 teaspoon salt
- 1 teaspoon cornstarch
- 1/2 cup honey
- 2 tablespoons lime juice
- 1/2 cup chicken stock
- 1 tablespoon water
- 4 tablespoons adobo sauce

For the Cauliflower Rice:

- 4 cups riced cauliflower
- 1/2 of red onion, peeled, chopped
- 1 lime, zested
- 1 medium red bell pepper, chopped
- 1/2 cup cilantro leaves
- 1/4 teaspoon salt
- 1 tablespoon lime juice
- 1 tablespoon olive oil

Method:

1. Switch on the oven, then set it to 375 degrees F, and let it preheat.
2. Meanwhile, prepare the meatballs and for this, place all its ingredients in a bowl, stir until well mixed and then shape the mixture into meatballs, each about 1 ½ tablespoon.
3. Take a baking sheet, line it with parchment sheet, place meatballs on it, and bake for 20 to 25 minutes until thoroughly cooked.
4. In the meantime, prepare the cauliflower rice and for this, take a skillet pan, place it over medium heat, add oil and when hot, add onion and bell pepper and cook for 4 minutes until slightly softened.
5. Then add cauliflower rice, season with salt and lime zest, stir well and continue cooking for 3 minutes until rice has softened slightly.

6. Add cilantro, drizzle with lime juice, stir well, then remove the pan from heat and set aside.
7. Then prepare the glaze and for this, take a saucepan, place all the ingredients For the glaze in it except for cornstarch and water, whisk until combined, and cook over medium heat for 3 minutes until hot.
8. Then stir together cornstarch and water, add to the saucepan, stir well and simmer the sauce until thickened slightly, stirring constantly.
9. Remove saucepan from heat, add meatballs in the sauce and toss until well coated, let cool until required.
10. For meal prep, divide cauliflower rice evenly between four heatproof meal prep containers, then add meatballs and drizzle with extra glaze.
11. Tighten the containers with lid and store in the refrigerator for up to four days or freeze for up to one month.
12. When ready to eat, thaw the meatballs, then reheat in the microwave until hot and serve.

Nutrition Value:

- Calories: 427 Cal
- Fat: 18 g
- Carbs: 47 g
- Protein: 26 g
- Fiber: 3 g

Lemon Butter Veggies and Sausage

Preparation time: 10 minutes
Cooking time: 35 minutes
Servings: 6

Ingredients:

- 4 medium carrots, peeled, diced
- 1½ pounds beef sausage, thickly sliced
- 2 medium red bell peppers, cored, diced
- 1 bunch of asparagus, cut into 1-inch pieces
- 1 bunch of radishes, halved
- 2 cups yellow cherry tomatoes
- 2 small zucchini, diced
- 1 small eggplant, diced
- 2 cups red cherry tomatoes
- 2/3 teaspoon ground black pepper
- 2 teaspoons salt

For the Lemon Butter:

- 1 tablespoon minced garlic
- 4 tablespoons butter, unsalted, melted
- 1 lemon, juiced, zested

Method:

1. Switch on the oven, then set it to 400 degrees F, and let it preheat.
2. Meanwhile, prepare the lemon butter and for this, place all its ingredients in a bowl and stir until combined.
3. Take a large baking sheet, place eggplant, carrots, bell pepper, and radish pieces in an even layer on it, then drizzle with half of the prepared lemon butter and toss well until coated.
4. Sprinkle vegetables with 1 teaspoon salt and ½ teaspoon black pepper and bake for 15 minutes until vegetables are just tender.
5. Then add remaining vegetables into the baking sheet along with sausage, drizzle with remaining lemon butter, season with remaining black pepper and salt, toss until combined and continue roasting for 20 minutes.
6. Let the vegetables and sausage cool completely, then divide evenly between six heatproof glass meal prep containers and tighten with lid.
7. Store the containers in the refrigerator for up to four days or freeze for up to one month.
8. When ready to eat, thaw the vegetables and sausage, then microwave until hot and serve.

Nutrition Value:

- Calories: 310 Cal
- Fat: 20 g
- Carbs: 18 g

- Protein: 16 g
- Fiber: 8 g

Steak and Garlic Roasted Potato

Preparation time: 10 minutes
Cooking time: 20 minutes
Servings: 2

Ingredients:

- 1/2 pound small white potatoes, peeled, sliced in quarters
- 1 cup broccoli florets, roasted
- 2 rib-eye steaks, each about 5 ounces
- 1 teaspoon garlic powder
- 1 teaspoon ground black pepper
- 1 ½ teaspoon salt
- 1 teaspoon dried thyme
- 3 tablespoons olive oil

Method:

1. Switch on the oven, then set it to 425 degrees F, and let it preheat.
2. Take a medium baking sheet, place potato slices on it, drizzle with 1 tablespoon oil, then sprinkle with garlic, black pepper, ½ teaspoon each of salt and thyme and bake for 20 minutes until tender.
3. Meanwhile, coat the steaks with remaining oil, then sprinkle remaining salt and black pepper on both sides and rub it into the steaks for 1 minute.
4. Place the griddle pan over medium heat and when hot, add steaks on it and grill for 5 minutes per side until cooked to medium level.
5. Let the steaks cool completely, then portion them between two heatproof meal prep containers and then evenly add potatoes and broccoli florets.
6. Tighten the containers with lid and refrigerate for up to four days or freeze for up to one month.
7. When ready to eat, thaw the steaks and vegetables, then microwave until hot and serve.

Nutrition Value:

- Calories: 461 Cal
- Fat: 29 g
- Carbs: 31 g
- Protein: 19 g
- Fiber: 18 g

Pulled Pork Taco Bowl

Preparation time: 5 minutes
Cooking time: 5 minutes
Servings: 4

Ingredients:

- 2 cups cooked pulled pork
- 4 tablespoons olive oil
- 1 cup chopped red onion
- 1 cup chopped red pepper
- 4 teaspoons taco seasoning
- 4 tablespoons water
- 4 jalapeno peppers, sliced
- 4 tablespoons lime juice
- 4 tablespoons chopped cilantro
- 8 tortillas, gluten-free

Method:

1. Take a skillet pan, place it over medium heat, add oil and when hot, add pork, onion, and red pepper, season with taco seasoning, drizzle with water, stir well and cook for 5 minutes until onions have softened.
2. Remove the pan from heat, then let the pork cool completely and portion evenly between four heatproof glass meal prep containers.
3. Garnish the pork with cilantro and jalapeno, drizzle 1 tablespoon lime juice on pork and then pack two tortillas separately in each container.
4. Tighten the container with the lid, and refrigerate for up to four days or freeze for up to one month.
5. When ready to eat, thaw the pork and then microwave until hot.
6. Assemble pork over the toasted tortilla and serve.

Nutrition Value:

- Calories: 248.6 Cal
- Fat: 5.3 g
- Carbs: 35.3 g
- Protein: 16 g
- Fiber: 4.2 g

Bean and Beef Slow-Cooked Chili

Preparation time: 10 minutes
Cooking time: 8 hours and 8 minutes
Servings: 6

Ingredients:

For the Chili:

- 1 pound ground beef
- 15 ounces cooked black beans
- 14-1/2 ounces diced tomatoes with green chilies
- 15 ounces cooked pinto beans
- 1 large sweet onion, peeled, chopped
- 1 ½ teaspoon minced garlic
- 1/2 teaspoon salt
- 2 teaspoons ground cumin
- 2 tablespoons red chili powder

For Serving:

- 4 tablespoons sour cream
- 4 tablespoons minced fresh cilantro

Method:

1. Take a large skillet pan, place it over medium heat and when hot, add beef, garlic, and onion and cook for 8 minutes until beef has nicely browned.
2. Transfer the beef into a slow cooker, top with half of the tomatoes, then add remaining ingredients, stir well and top with remaining tomatoes.
3. Switch on the slow cooker, then shut it with the lid and cook for 8 hours at a low heat setting until the chili has thoroughly cooked.
4. Let the chili cool, then portion it evenly between four heatproof meal prep containers, tighten with lid, and freeze for up to one month.
5. When ready to eat, thaw the chili, microwave until hot, and then top with 1 tablespoon sour cream and cilantro and serve.

Nutrition Value:

- Calories: 370.1 Cal
- Fat: 12.9 g
- Carbs: 43 g
- Protein: 23.2 g
- Fiber: 15 g

Garlic Peppered Steak

Preparation time: 10 minutes
Cooking time: 40 minutes
Servings: 4

Ingredients:

- 2 pounds flank steak

For the Seasonings:

- ¼ teaspoon sea salt
- 1 tablespoon minced garlic
- 1 1/2 tablespoon red pepper flakes
- 1 1/2 tablespoon smoked paprika
- 2 tablespoons ground black pepper
- 2 tablespoons olive oil

For Serving:

- 2 cups cooked brown rice
- 4 tablespoons lime juice
- 4 tablespoons chopped parsley

Method:

1. Switch on the oven, then set it to 275 degrees F, and let it preheat.
2. Meanwhile, coat the top of flank steaks with oil, then sprinkle with all the seasonings and rub into the meat for 1 minute.
3. Place the steak in the baking sheet and roast for 35 to 40 minutes until steak is cooked to the desired level, flipping halfway through.
4. Let steaks cool slightly, then evenly portion between four heatproof glass meal prep bowls, add brown rice, tighten with lid, and freeze for up to one month.
5. When ready to eat, thaw the steaks and rice, microwave until hot, then garnish with parsley, drizzle with lime juice and serve.

Nutrition Value:

- Calories: 377 Cal
- Fat: 13 g
- Carbs: 27 g
- Protein: 38 g
- Fiber: 12 g

Burger and Veggie Bowls

Preparation time: 10 minutes
Cooking time: 15 minutes
Servings: 4

Ingredients:

For the Burgers:

- 1 pound ground beef
- 1 teaspoon garlic powder
- 1 teaspoon salt
- ½ teaspoon ground black pepper
- ½ teaspoon paprika
- 1 teaspoon dried thyme
- 2 tablespoons olive oil
- 1 egg

For the Vegetables:

- 2 zucchini, sliced
- 1 medium butternut squash, peeled, diced
- 2 cups cherry tomatoes halves
- ½ teaspoon salt
- ¼ teaspoon ground black pepper
- 4 tablespoons olive oil

Method:

1. Switch on the oven, then set it to 425 degrees F, and let it preheat.
2. Take a baking sheet, place zucchini and butternut squash on it, season with salt and black pepper, toss until well coated roasted for 15 minutes until vegetables are tender.
3. Meanwhile, prepare the burger and for this, place all its ingredients in a bowl, mix well and then shape into four thick patties.
4. Take a grill pan, place it over medium heat, grease it with oil and when hot, add patties and cook for 5 minutes per side until thoroughly cooked.
5. Let the vegetables and patties cool, then portion them evenly between four heatproof glass meal prep containers and tighten with lid.
6. When ready to eat, thaw the burgers and vegetables and then reheat in the microwave oven until hot.
7. Serve with cherry tomatoes.

Nutrition Value:

- Calories: 280 Cal
- Fat: 8 g
- Carbs: 16 g
- Protein: 36 g
- Fiber: 7 g

Chili Beef Pasta

Preparation time: 10 minutes
Cooking time: 30 minutes
Servings: 4

Ingredients:

- 8 ounces spiral pasta, gluten-free, uncooked
- 1 pound ground beef
- 2 tablespoons minced onion, dried
- 1/2 teaspoon garlic powder
- 2 teaspoons red chili powder
- 2 teaspoons dried oregano
- 1 teaspoon sugar
- 1/8 teaspoon salt
- 6 ounces tomato paste
- 2 cups water
- 3 cups tomato juice

Method:

1. Take a large saucepan, place it over medium heat and when hot, add beef and cook for 8 minutes until beef is no longer pink.
2. Drain the excess fat from the pan, add remaining ingredients except for pasta, stir well and bring the mixture to boil.
3. Then reduce heat to medium-low level, add pasta and simmer for 20 minutes until pasta is tender, covering the pan.
4. Remove the saucepan from heat, let the pasta cool completely and then portion it evenly between four heatproof glass meal prep containers.
5. Tighten the containers with lid and store in the freezer for up to one month.
6. When ready to eat, thaw the pasta, then reheat in the microwave oven until hot and serve.

Nutrition Value:

- Calories: 312 Cal
- Fat: 7 g
- Carbs: 43 g
- Protein: 20 g
- Fiber: 3 g

Beef and Pepper Stew

Preparation time: 10 minutes
Cooking time: 35 minutes
Servings: 4

Ingredients:

- 2 cups instant rice, uncooked
- 1 pound ground beef
- 44 ounces diced tomatoes
- 1 large white onion, peeled, chopped
- 4 large green bell peppers, cored, chopped
- 8 ounces chopped green chilies
- 3 teaspoons garlic powder
- 1 teaspoon ground black pepper
- 1/4 teaspoon salt

Method:

1. Place a large saucepan over medium heat and when hot, add beef and cook for 8 minutes until beef is no longer pink.
2. Add remaining ingredients except for rice and bring the mixture to boil.
3. Then reduce the heat to the medium-low level and simmer the stew for 25 minutes until vegetables are tender.
4. Meanwhile, prepare the rice, and for this, cook them according to instructions on their package.
5. When done, let stew and rice cool completely, then portion evenly between four heatproof glass meal prep containers.
6. Tighten the containers with lid and store in the freezer for up to one month.
7. When ready to eat, thaw the stew, then reheat in the microwave oven until hot and serve.

Nutrition Value:

- Calories: 244 Cal
- Fat: 5 g
- Carbs: 35 g
- Protein: 15 g
- Fiber: 5 g

Beef Ragu Pasta

Preparation time: 10 minutes
Cooking time: 9 hours
Servings: 8

Ingredients:

- 28-ounce crushed tomatoes
- 1 ½ pound sirloin roast
- 1 medium white onion, peeled, chopped
- 2 medium carrots, peeled, chopped
- 1 teaspoon sliced garlic
- 1 teaspoon ground black pepper
- 1 ½ teaspoon salt
- 1 teaspoon dried thyme
- 3 dried bay leaves
- 1 tablespoon olive oil
- 1 cup beef broth
- 1 pound pasta, gluten-free, uncooked

Method:

1. Coat roast with oil, then season with salt and black pepper on both sides and rub the seasonings into the meat for 1 minute.
2. Then place steaks into a slow cooker, top with tomatoes, add onion, carrots, garlic, thyme, bay leaf and pour in broth.
3. Switch on the slow cooker, shut it with lid and cook for 6 hours at high heat setting or 9 hours at low heat setting.
4. Meanwhile, prepare the pasta and for this, place a pot over medium heat half-full with water and bring it to boil.
5. Then add pasta, cook for 10 minutes until tender, then drain it and set aside until required.
6. When done, remove bay leaf, shred the beef, stir well and let cool completely.
7. Portion beef evenly between eight heatproof glass meal prep containers, add pasta, then tighten the containers with lid and store in the freezer for up to one month.
8. When ready to eat, thaw the beef and pasta, then reheat in the microwave oven until hot and serve.

Nutrition Value:

- Calories: 444 Cal
- Fat: 12 g
- Carbs: 44 g
- Protein: 40 g
- Fiber: 23 g

Orange-Sage Pork Chops

Preparation time: 10 minutes
Cooking time: 12 minutes
Servings: 4

Ingredients:

- 4 pork chops, boneless, each about 5 ounces
- ½ teaspoon ground black pepper
- 1 1/4 teaspoon cornstarch
- ½ teaspoon salt
- ½ teaspoon minced garlic
- 1 teaspoon orange zest
- 3 tablespoons butter
- 2 teaspoons honey
- 1 1/2 teaspoon lemon juice
- 1/4 cup orange juice, unsweetened
- 1/4 cup chicken broth
- 2 teaspoons chopped fresh sage leaves

Method:

1. Prepare the pork chops, and for this, season them with salt and black pepper.
2. Take a skillet pan, place it over medium-high heat, add 2 tablespoons butter and when it melts, add pork chops and cook for 4 minutes per side until a meat thermometer inserted into the thickest part of pork reads 145 degrees F.
3. Transfer pork chops to a plate and let them rest.
4. Place cornstarch in a small bowl and whisk in honey, lemon juice, orange juice, and broth until smooth.
5. Reduce the heat to medium level, add the remaining butter in the pan and when it melts, add garlic and cook for 20 seconds until fragrant.
6. Pour in orange juice mixture, stir well and bring the mixture to boil, whisking constantly.
7. Reduce heat to the low level, simmer the sauce for 1 minute, add sage and orange zest and stir until mixed, remove the pan from heat and let the sauce cool.
8. Portion pork chops evenly between four heatproof glass meal prep containers, drizzle with sauce on top, then tighten the containers with lid and store in the freezer for up to one month.
9. When ready to eat, thaw the pork, then reheat in the microwave oven until hot and serve with boiled brown rice and green salad.

Nutrition Value:

- Calories: 182 Cal
- Fat: 9.4 g
- Carbs: 5.6 g
- Protein: 18.4 g
- Fiber: 1.1 g

Steak Fajitas

Preparation time: 15 minutes
Cooking time: 15 minutes
Servings: 4

Ingredients:

For the Fajita Seasoning:

- 1 teaspoon onion powder
- 1 teaspoon garlic powder
- 1/2 teaspoon sea salt
- 1 teaspoon cumin
- 2 teaspoons red chili powder
- 1 teaspoon smoked paprika

For the Fajitas:

- 2 medium green bell peppers, cored, sliced into strips
- 1 ½ pounds flank steak
- 2 medium red bell peppers, cored, sliced into strips
- 1 medium red onion, peeled, sliced into strips
- 2 limes, juiced
- 1 tablespoon Worcestershire sauce
- 3 tablespoons olive oil
- 2 tablespoons butter, unsalted

For Serving:

- 2 cups cooked cauliflower rice

Method:

1. Prepare the seasoning and for this, place all its ingredients in a bowl and stir well until mixed, set aside until required.
2. Prepare fajitas and for this, place 5 teaspoons of fajita seasoning in a small bowl, add 2 tablespoon oil, mustard, lemon juice, whisk until combined, and then pour the mixture in a large plastic bag.
3. Add steak, seal the bag, turn the bag upside down to coat steak with fajita mixture and let it rest for 10 minutes.
4. Meanwhile, take a large pan, place it over medium-high heat, add 1 tablespoon oil and hot, add onions, cook for 4 minutes until softened, then add bell peppers and sprinkle with remaining fajita seasoning.
5. Continue cooking for 3 minutes until peppers are tender-crisp, then transfer vegetables to a plate and set aside.
6. Add butter in the skillet pan, then add steaks and cook for 4 minutes per side or more until cooked to the desired level.

7. Then transfer steaks to a cutting board, let them cool for 10 minutes and then cut into slice strips.
8. Portion steaks evenly between four heatproof glass meal prep containers, add vegetables and cauliflower rice, then tighten the containers with lid and store in the freezer for up to one month.
9. When ready to eat, thaw the steaks, then reheat in the microwave oven until hot and serve.

Nutrition Value:

- Calories: 532 Cal
- Fat: 38 g
- Carbs: 11 g
- Protein: 36 g
- Fiber: 3 g

Chapter 8: Vegetarian

Bean Salad

Preparation time: 10 minutes
Cooking time: 0 minutes
Servings: 4

Ingredients:

For the Salad:

- 16 ounces cooked kidney beans
- 3 cups cooked basmati rice
- 15 ounces cooked black beans
- 1/4 cup minced cilantro
- 1 1/2 cups frozen corn, thawed
- 4 green onions, sliced
- 1 small sweet red pepper, chopped

For the Dressing:

- ½ teaspoon minced garlic
- 1 teaspoon red chili powder
- 1 teaspoon salt
- 1/4 teaspoon ground black pepper
- 1 teaspoon ground cumin
- 1 tablespoon coconut sugar
- 1/2 cup olive oil
- 1/4 cup apple cider vinegar

Method:

1. Prepare the dressing and for this, place all its ingredients in a small bowl and whisk until combined.
2. Place all the ingredients For the salad in another bowl, drizzle with salad dressing and toss until well coated.
3. Portion the salad evenly between four salad mason jars and tighten with lid.
4. Store the salad in the refrigerator for up to three days and serve.

Nutrition Value:

- Calories: 440 Cal
- Fat: 19 g
- Carbs: 58 g
- Protein: 12 g
- Fiber: 8 g

Quinoa and Black Bean Stuffed Peppers

Preparation time: 15 minutes
Cooking time: 20 minutes
Servings: 4

Ingredients:

- 4 large green bell peppers
- 1 cup quinoa, uncooked
- 15 ounces cooked black beans
- 1/2 cup ricotta cheese
- 2 cups tomato salsa
- 1/2 cup shredded Monterey Jack cheese
- 1 1/2 cups water

Method:

1. Switch on the oven, then set it to 400 degrees F, and let preheat.
2. Take a small saucepan, place it over medium heat, pour in water, bring it boil, then add quinoa, reduce heat to medium-low level and simmer for 10 minutes until the quinoa has absorbed all the liquid.
3. Meanwhile, prepare the peppers and for this, cut the peppers from the top, and remove seeds from them.
4. Take an 8 inches baking dish, grease it with oil, place peppers in it cut side down and microwave for 4 minutes until tender-crisp.
5. When quinoa has cooked, fluff it with a fork, then add 1 2/3 cups salsa along with ¼ cup Jack cheese, ricotta cheese, and beans and stir until well combined.
6. Turn the bell pepper in the baking pan, cut side up, then stuff with the quinoa mixture, sprinkle remaining Jack cheese on top of stuffed peppers, and bake for 15 minutes.
7. Let the peppers cool completely, then portion between four heatproof glass meal prep containers, tighten the container with lid and store in the refrigerator for up to one week or freeze for up to two months.
8. When ready to eat, thaw the peppers, then reheat in the microwave until hot, top with remaining salsa and serve.

Nutrition Value:

- Calories: 393 Cal
- Fat: 8 g
- Carbs: 59 g
- Protein: 18 g
- Fiber: 10 g

Moroccan Chickpea Quinoa Salad

Preparation time: 10 minutes
Cooking time: 22 minutes
Servings: 4

Ingredients:

- 15 ounces cooked chickpeas
- 1 cup quinoa, uncooked
- 1 medium white onion, peeled, diced
- ⅔ cup dried cranberries
- ⅓ cup diced parsley
- ½ teaspoon cumin
- ¼ teaspoon ground black pepper
- 1/2 teaspoon salt
- ½ teaspoon cinnamon
- 1 teaspoon ground turmeric
- ½ tablespoon coconut oil
- 2 cups vegetarian broth
- ½ cup sliced toasted almonds

Method:

1. Take a large pot, place it over medium heat, add oil and when hot, add onion and cook for 5 minutes until sauté.
2. Then season with salt, black pepper, cumin, turmeric, and cinnamon and continue cooking for 30 seconds until fragrant.
3. Add quinoa into the pot, pour in the broth, stir well and bring the mixture to boil.
4. Then reduce heat to the low level and simmer the quinoa for 15 minutes until all the liquid is absorbed, covering the pot.
5. Remove the pot from heat, let it rest for 5 minutes, then fluff the quinoa with a fork, add chickpeas, parsley and cranberries and stir until well combined.
6. Let the salad cool completely, then evenly portion between four salad mason jars and top with almonds.
7. Tighten the jars with lid and refrigerate the salad for up to three days.
8. Serve straight away.

Nutrition Value:

- Calories: 448 Cal
- Fat: 13.8 g
- Carbs: 70.2 g
- Protein: 16.5 g
- Fiber: 12.7 g

Sweet Potato and Lentil Salads

Preparation time: 15 minutes
Cooking time: 25 minutes
Servings: 4

Ingredients:

For the Vinaigrette:

- 1 tablespoon minced garlic
- 1/2 teaspoon red chili powder
- 1/4 teaspoon salt
- 2 teaspoons honey
- 2 teaspoons lime juice
- 2 tablespoons apple cider vinegar
- 2 tablespoons olive oil

For the Salad:

- 19 ounces cooked brown lentils
- 6 cups sweet potato cubes
- 1 red bell pepper, sliced
- 11.5 ounces cooked corn kernels
- 1/2 teaspoon red chili powder
- 1 tablespoon olive oil

Method:

1. Switch on the oven, then set it to 425 degrees F, and let preheat.
2. Prepare the vinaigrette and for this, place all its ingredients in a shaker and shake until well combined, set aside until required.
3. Take a baking sheet, place sweet potato on it, drizzle with oil, toss until well coated, season with red chili powder and bake for 25 minutes until roasted, stirring halfway through, and when done, the sweet potato cubes cool completely.
4. Assemble the salad and for this, spoon 1 tablespoon of prepared vinaigrette in four salad mason jars, then add ½ cup cooked lentils into each jar, top with ½ cup corn, 1 cup sweet potato, and slices of red bell pepper.
5. Tighten the mason jars with lid and store in the refrigerator for up to four days.

Nutrition Value:

- Calories: 416 Cal
- Fat: 12 g
- Carbs: 66 g
- Protein: 13 g
- Fiber: 13 g

Orange Tofu Chickpea Bowls

Preparation time: 10 minutes
Cooking time: 15 minutes
Servings: 4

Ingredients:

- 14 ounces tofu, pressed, drained, cubed
- 6 cups broccoli florets, steamed
- 2 cups cooked brown rice
- 12 ounces cooked chickpeas
- 2 teaspoons sesame oil
- 1 tablespoon tamari
- 2 teaspoons sesame seeds

For the Orange Sauce:

- ½ teaspoon minced garlic
- 2 tablespoons maple syrup
- 1/2 teaspoon grated ginger
- 2 teaspoons cornstarch
- 2 tablespoons tamari
- 2 tablespoons toasted sesame oil
- 1/2 cup orange juice, unsweetened
- 1/4 cup water

Method:

1. Prepare the sauce and for this, place all its ingredients in a small bowl and whisk until well combined.
2. Take a large skillet pan, place it over medium heat, add sesame oil and when hot, add tofu, drizzle with tamari and cook for 7 to 10 minutes until nicely browned.
3. Then add chickpeas, pour in orange juice, stir well and cook for 3 minutes until the sauce has thickened enough to coat the back of a spoon, let cool completely.
4. For meal prep, evenly portion rice between four heatproof glass meal prep containers, then add ¼ of the steamed broccoli into each container, top with ¼ of orange tofu and chickpeas, drizzle with extra sauce and garnish with sesame seeds.
5. Tighten the containers with lid and refrigerate for up to five days or freeze for up to one month.
6. When ready to eat, reheat the container in the microwave until hot and serve.

Nutrition Value:

- Calories: 348 Cal
- Fat: 9 g
- Carbs: 45 g
- Protein: 20 g
- Fiber: 12 g

Tofu Stir Fry

Preparation time: 15 minutes
Cooking time: 28 minutes
Servings: 3

Ingredients:

- 1 bunch of baby bok choy, rinsed
- 1 ½ cups cooked brown rice
- 14 ounces tofu, pressed, drained, cubed
- 1 medium head of broccoli, chopped
- 3 medium carrots, peeled, chopped
- ½ teaspoon ground black pepper
- 1 teaspoon salt
- 3 tablespoons olive oil
- 1 teaspoon soy sauce
- 1 tablespoon water

For the Peanut Sauce:

- ½ teaspoon minced garlic
- 1/4 cup honey
- 1/4 cup soy sauce
- 1 teaspoon apple cider vinegar
- 1/4 cup peanut butter
- 1 teaspoon sesame oil

Method:

1. Switch on the oven, then set it to 400 degrees F, and let it preheat.
2. Meanwhile, prepare the sauce and for this, place all its ingredients in a large bowl and whisk until combined.
3. Add tofu cubes in the sauce, toss until well coated and set aside.
4. Take a large skillet pan, place it over medium heat, add 1 tablespoon oil and when hot, add bok choy, season with salt and black pepper and cook for 5 minutes.
5. Then portion bok choy into three heatproof glass meal prep containers and set aside until required.
6. Add 1 tablespoon oil in the pan, add broccoli and carrot, sprinkle with black pepper, drizzle with soy sauce and water, stir well and cook for 7 minutes, covering the pan.
7. Then portion the vegetables into meal prep containers containing bok choy and set aside until required.
8. Add remaining oil into the skillet pan, add tofu pieces in it and cook for 10 minutes until nicely browned, flipping the tofu every 3 minutes.
9. Take a baking sheet, line it with aluminum foil, spread tofu pieces on it, and bake for 5 minutes.

10. Add ½ cup cooked brown rice into each meal prep container, then top with tofu, let cool completely, and then tighten the container with lid.
11. Store the meal prep container in the refrigerator for up to four days or freeze for up to two months.
12. When ready to eat, reheat the container in the microwave until hot and serve.

Nutrition Value:

- Calories: 272.2 Cal
- Fat: 8.4 g
- Carbs: 34.2 g
- Protein: 15.1 g
- Fiber: 10.8 g

Grilled Vegetable and Black Bean Bowls

Preparation time: 10 minutes
Cooking time: 15 minutes
Servings: 4

Ingredients:

For the Vinaigrette:

- 1/4 teaspoon salt
- 1/4 teaspoon red chili powder
- 2 teaspoons honey
- 2 tablespoons apple cider vinegar
- 3 tablespoons BBQ sauce
- 1 teaspoon lime juice

For the Meal Prep Bowls:

- 2 cups cooked quinoa
- 18 ounces cooked black beans
- 1 medium zucchini, chopped
- ½ of medium red onion, peeled, chopped
- 2 medium red bell peppers, chopped
- 2/3 teaspoon ground black pepper
- 1 teaspoon salt
- 1 tablespoon olive oil

Method:

1. Prepare the vinaigrette, and for this, place all its ingredients in a shaker and shale until well combined, set aside until required.
2. Place zucchini, onion and bell pepper in a large bowl, drizzle with oil, season with black pepper and salt, and toss until well coated.
3. Take a grill pan, place it over medium heat, grease it with oil and when hot, arrange vegetables on it and grill for 10 to 15 minutes until cooked, flipping every 5 minutes.
4. For meal prep, portion quinoa into four heatproof glass meal prep containers, top evenly with grilled vegetables and black pepper, and then drizzle with vinaigrette generously.
5. Tighten the meal prep containers with lid and store in the refrigerator for up to four days or freeze for up to two months.
6. When ready to eat, reheat the container in the microwave until hot, and serve.

Nutrition Value:

- Calories: 329 Cal
- Fat: 6 g
- Carbs: 56 g
- Protein: 14 g
- Fiber: 11 g

Roasted Tomatoes and Mushrooms

Preparation time: 10 minutes
Cooking time: 35 minutes
Servings: 4

Ingredients:

- 2 cups cooked quinoa
- 4 cups cherry tomatoes, halved
- 1 pound small cremini mushrooms, halved
- 2 tablespoons minced garlic
- 2 tablespoons fresh thyme leaves
- 1/2 teaspoon ground black pepper
- 1/2 teaspoon salt
- 1 tablespoon apple cider vinegar
- 3 tablespoons olive oil

Method:

1. Switch on the oven, then set it to 375 degrees F, and let it preheat.
2. Place cherry tomatoes in a large bowl, drizzle with 1 tablespoon oil, season with ¼ teaspoon each of salt and black pepper, sprinkle with 1 tablespoon thyme and toss until combined.
3. Take a large rimmed baking sheet and arrange tomatoes on its one half, cut-side down, and spread in the single layer.
4. Place mushrooms in the same bowl, add garlic, drizzle with remaining oil, season with remaining salt, thyme and black pepper, and toss until combined.
5. Transfer the mushrooms to the other half of the baking sheet, spread them in a single layer, and bake for 30 to 35 minutes until tomatoes and mushrooms are softened and caramelized.
6. Mash the tomatoes with a fork, then drizzle vinegar over the vegetables and toss until well combined.
7. For meal prep, take four heatproof glass meal prep containers, add ½ cup of quinoa into each container and then top evenly with tomato and mushroom mixture.
8. Tighten the container with lid and store them in the refrigerator for up to four days.
9. When ready to eat, reheat the container in the microwave until hot and serve.

Nutrition Value:

- Calories: 160 Cal
- Fat: 10.7 g
- Carbs: 15 g
- Protein: 5 g
- Fiber: 3.6 g

Chapter 9: Fish and Seafood

Honey Lemon Salmon and Broccolini

Preparation time: 15 minutes
Cooking time: 15 minutes
Servings: 4

Ingredients:

- 4 salmon fillets, each about 5 ounces
- 12 ounces Broccolini
- 1 teaspoon ground black pepper
- 1 teaspoon salt
- 2 tablespoons olive oil
- 2 teaspoons sesame seeds

For the Honey Lemon Sauce:

- 1 teaspoon minced garlic
- 2 teaspoons cornstarch
- 2 tablespoons soy sauce
- 1/4 cup honey
- 1 tablespoon sesame oil
- 1 lemon, juiced
- 1/4 cup water

Method:

1. Switch on the oven, then set it to 425 degrees F, and let it preheat.
2. Place salmon in a large sheet pan, brush it with olive oil, add Broccolini, toss it oil until coated, then season with salt and black pepper and bake for 10 minutes.
3. In the meantime, prepare the sauce and for this, place all its ingredients in a shaker and shake until well combined, and no clumps remain in the sauce.
4. When salmon and Broccolini has roasted, drizzle the sauce on them, return the sheet pan into the oven, switch on the broiler and continue cooking for 3 to 5 minutes until salmon and Broccolini are nicely browned, rotating the sheet pan halfway through.
5. Let the salmon and Broccolini cool, then portion evenly between four heatproof glass meal prep container and garnish with sesame seeds.
6. Tighten the containers with lid and refrigerate for up to four days or freeze for up to one month.
7. When ready to eat, thaw the salmon, then reheat the container in the microwave until hot and serve with boiled brown rice.

Nutrition Value:

- Calories: 345 Cal
- Fat: 12 g
- Carbs: 27 g
- Protein: 34 g
- Fiber: 1 g

Tuna Cakes

Preparation time: 15 minutes
Cooking time: 16 minutes
Servings: 12

Ingredients:

- 24 ounces cooked tuna
- 3/4 cup almond flour
- 1 small onion, peeled, diced
- 2 tablespoons chopped parsley
- 1/4 cup scallions, chopped
- 1/4 cup roasted red peppers, chopped
- 1/2 teaspoon ground black pepper
- 1 teaspoon salt
- 1 teaspoon minced garlic
- 1/2 teaspoon lemon zest
- 1/2 teaspoon paprika
- 1 teaspoon lemon juice
- 1 teaspoon Sriracha sauce
- 1 egg
- 1 egg white

For Roasted Red Pepper Sauce:

- 1 cup roasted red pepper
- 3 cloves of garlic, peeled
- 2 tablespoon chopped parsley
- 1/4 teaspoon ground black pepper
- 1/2 teaspoon sea salt
- 1/2 teaspoon cumin
- 1/2 teaspoon smoked paprika
- 1 1/2 tablespoon lemon juice
- 1/4 cup mayonnaise

Method:

1. Prepare the tuna cakes and for this, place all its ingredients in a large bowl, stir until well combined, and then shape the mixture into ¾ inch thick patties, about ¼ cup of the tuna mixture per patty.
2. Take a large skillet, grease it with oil and when hot, add tuna cakes in a single layer and cook for 4 minutes until side until nicely browned on both sides.
3. Transfer the tuna cakes to a plate and cook the remaining tuna cakes in the same manner, let cool completely.
4. Prepare the sauce, and for this, place all its ingredients in a blender and pulse until smooth.
5. Portion the cakes evenly between four heatproof glass meal prep containers and then portion the sauce separately in the containers.
6. Tighten the containers with lid and store in the refrigerator for up to four days or freeze for up to two months.

Nutrition Value:

- Calories: 251 Cal
- Fat: 12.6 g
- Carbs: 7.2 g
- Protein: 27 g
- Fiber: 1.8 g

Tuna Salad Lettuce Wraps

Preparation time: 15 minutes
Cooking time: 0 minute
Servings: 4

Ingredients:

For the Salad:

- 8 ounces cooked tuna
- 1 shallot bulb, peeled, diced
- 1/2 dill pickle, diced
- 1 rib of celery, peeled, diced
- 1/4 teaspoon garlic powder
- 1/4 teaspoon sea salt
- 1/4 teaspoon ground black pepper
- 1 tablespoon Dijon mustard
- 2 tablespoons lemon juice
- 2 tablespoons mayonnaise
- 2 tablespoons Greek yogurt

For Serving:

- 6 large romaine lettuce leaves, rinsed
- 2 cups grapes
- 2 medium carrots, peeled, cut into thin strips
- 2 medium cucumbers, cut into thin strips

Method:

1. Place tuna in a bowl, shred it with two forks, then add remaining ingredients and stir until well combined.
2. Portion carrots, cucumber, and grapes into four heatproof glass meal prep containers, then portion 2 large lettuce leaves into each container and top with 2/3 cup of tuna salad.
3. Tighten the containers with lid and refrigerate for up to four days.
4. Serve straight away.

Nutrition Value:

- Calories: 320 Cal
- Fat: 14 g
- Carbs: 23 g
- Protein: 29 g
- Fiber: 13 g

Cod and Veggies

Preparation time: 10 minutes
Cooking time: 25 minutes
Servings: 4

Ingredients:

- 1 pound cod, cut into 4 pieces
- 2 cups cherry tomatoes
- 2 cups diced purple potatoes
- 1 teaspoon dried thyme
- 1 ½ teaspoon salt
- 1 teaspoon ground black pepper
- 1 teaspoon garlic powder
- 4 tablespoons olive oil

Method:

1. Switch on the oven, then set it to 400 degrees F, and let it preheat.
2. Take a baking sheet, spread potatoes on it, drizzle with 2 tablespoons oil, toss until well coated, and roast for 15 minutes.
3. Then add push tomatoes to one side of the sheet, add cod and tomatoes, drizzle remaining oil over them, season with black pepper, salt, thyme, and garlic powder and then continue baking for 10 minutes until thoroughly cooked.
4. Let the salmon, potatoes, and tomatoes cool and then portion evenly between four heatproof meal prep containers.
5. Tighten the containers with lid and store in the refrigerator for up to four days or freeze for up to one month.
6. When ready to eat, thaw the fish and vegetables, then reheat in a microwave until hot and serve.

Nutrition Value:

- Calories: 267 Cal
- Fat: 11 g
- Carbs: 19 g
- Protein: 23 g
- Fiber: 9 g

Salad with Chickpeas and Tuna

Preparation time: 10 minutes
Cooking time: 0 minutes
Servings: 1

Ingredients:

- 2.5-ounce tuna, pouched
- ½ cup cooked chickpeas
- 3 cups chopped kale
- 1 medium carrot, peeled and shredded
- 2 tablespoons honey-mustard vinaigrette

Method:

1. Cut kale into bite-size pieces, add them in a bowl, then add vinaigrette and toss until well coated.
2. Transfer kale into a 1-quart mason jar, top with chickpeas, tuna, and carrot and tighten the jar with lid.
3. Refrigerate the jar for up to two days and serve.

Nutrition Value:

- Calories: 430 Cal
- Fat: 23 g
- Carbs: 30 g
- Protein: 26 g
- Fiber: 8 g

Shrimp Avocado Salad

Preparation time: 10 minutes
Cooking time: 0 minutes
Servings: 6

Ingredients:

For the Salad:

- 1 pound shrimp, peeled, deveined, cooked, chopped
- 1/4 cup chopped red onion
- 2 plum tomatoes, seeded, chopped
- 1 jalapeno pepper, deseeded, minced
- 2 green onions, chopped
- 1 serrano pepper, deseeded, minced
- 2 tablespoons minced fresh cilantro

For the Dressing:

- 1 teaspoon adobo seasoning
- 2 tablespoons apple cider vinegar
- 2 tablespoons lime juice
- 2 tablespoons olive oil

For Serving:

- 3 medium avocados, peeled and cubed
- 12 big lettuce leaves
- 6 wedges of lime

Method:

1. Place all the ingredients for the salad in a large bowl and toss until just mixed.
2. Prepare the dressing and for this, place all its ingredients in a small bowl and whisk until combined.
3. Drizzle the dressing over the salad, toss until well coated, and then stir in avocado.
4. Portion two lettuce leaves into six heatproof glass meal prep containers, then top evenly with prepared salad.
5. Add a lime wedge into each container, then tighten the containers with lid and store in the refrigerator for up to three days.
6. Serve straight away as a wrap.

Nutrition Value:

- Calories: 252 Cal
- Fat: 16 g
- Carbs: 11 g
- Protein: 17 g
- Fiber: 5 g

Tuna and White Bean Salad

Preparation time: 10 minutes
Cooking time: 0 minutes
Servings: 2

Ingredients:

For the Salad:

- 15 ounces cooked cannellini beans
- 8 ounces cooked tuna
- 1/3 cup chopped roasted sweet red peppers
- 4 cups fresh arugula
- 1/2 of small red onion, peeled, sliced
- 1 cup grape tomatoes, halved
- 1/3 cup pitted olives
- 1/4 cup chopped fresh basil

For the Dressing:

- ½ teaspoon minced garlic
- 1/2 teaspoon grated lemon zest
- 1/8 teaspoon salt
- 3 tablespoons olive oil
- 2 tablespoons lemon juice

Method:

1. Prepare the salad dressing and for this, place all its ingredients in a bowl and whisk until combined.
2. Take two mason jars, spoon the dressing evenly in its bottom, evenly portion tomatoes, olives, onion, arugula, and red pepper, then top with beans and tuna and tighten the jars with lid.
3. Refrigerate the jars for up to three days and serve.

Nutrition Value:

- Calories: 319 Cal
- Fat: 16 g
- Carbs: 20 g
- Protein: 23 g
- Fiber: 5 g

Lime Shrimp Zoodles

Preparation time: 10 minutes
Cooking time: 10 minutes
Servings: 4

Ingredients:

- 6 cups spiralized zucchini
- 1 pound uncooked shrimp, peeled, deveined
- 1 medium shallot, peeled, minced
- 1 teaspoon minced garlic
- 1/2 teaspoon ground black pepper
- 1/2 teaspoon salt
- 1 1/2 teaspoons grated lime zest
- 1 tablespoon olive oil
- 3 tablespoons butter, unsalted
- 2 tablespoons lime juice
- 1/4 cup tequila
- 1/4 cup minced fresh parsley

Method:

1. Take a large skillet, place it over medium heat, add 2 tablespoons butter and when it melts, add garlic and shallots and cook for 2 minutes.
2. Remove the pan from heat, add tequila, lime juice, and zest and stir until mixed.
3. Return the pan over medium heat and continue cooking for 3 minutes until all the liquid in the pan has evaporated.
4. Add remaining butter into the pan, along with butter, add shrimps and zucchini, season with salt and black pepper, stir well and cook for 5 minutes until shrimps have thoroughly cooked.
5. Let the shrimps and zucchini cool, then portion between four heatproof glass meal prep containers and garnish with parsley.
6. Tighten the containers with lid and refrigerate for up to four days or freeze for up to one month.
7. When ready to eat, reheat the containers in the microwave and serve.

Nutrition Value:

- Calories: 246 Cal
- Fat: 14 g
- Carbs: 7 g
- Protein: 20 g
- Fiber: 1 g

Chapter 10: Desserts

Collagen Brownie Cups

Preparation time: 1 hour and 10 minutes
Cooking time: 1 minute
Servings: 12

Ingredients:

- 1/4 cup almond flour
- 1/2 cup collagen peptides
- 1/4 cup cocoa powder, unsweetened
- 1 cup chocolate chips
- 1/4 cup peanut butter
- 3 tablespoons maple syrup
- 1/2 cup almond milk, unsweetened

Method:

1. Place 2/3 cup chocolate chips in a heatproof bowl and microwave for 30 seconds until chocolate has melted.
2. Take a 12 cups mini muffin pan, line its cups with muffin liner, then fill each cup with 1 tablespoon of melted chocolate, swirling it with the back of a spoon and then freeze for 30 minutes until set.
3. Meanwhile, prepare the filling and for this, place the remaining ingredients in a bowl and mix well until sticky dough comes together.
4. Shape the dough into balls and then flatten each ball into discs.
5. When the chocolate has set, place dough disc into each muffin cup and then flatten it by using fingers to press the disc against the sides of muffin cup.
6. Place remaining chocolate chips in a heatproof bowl, microwave for 30 seconds until chocolate has melted, then evenly pour the chocolate on dough crust until covered and freeze for another 30 minutes until set.
7. Then transfer the cups in a large plastic bag and store in the freezer for up to three months.

Nutrition Value:

- Calories: 182 Cal
- Fat: 9.5 g
- Carbs: 19.8 g
- Protein: 6.4 g
- Fiber: 2.6 g

Chocolate Almond Bark

Preparation time: 1 hour and 10 minutes
Cooking time: 2 minutes
Servings: 4

Ingredients:

- 1 3/4 cup cacao
- 1/4 cup slivered almonds, unsalted
- 1 tablespoon erythritol sweetener
- 1/4 cup almond butter, unsweetened

Method:

1. Place cacao in a heatproof bowl, add butter and sweetener and microwave for 1 to 2 minutes until cacao and butter have melted, stirring every 30 seconds.
2. Take a baking sheet, line it with parchment sheet, then pour the cacao mixture on it and spread it evenly with the back of a spoon.
3. Sprinkle almond on top of cacao mixture and then freeze for 1 hour until hard.
4. Then break it into pieces, place the pieces in a large plastic bag, and store in the freezer for up to three months.

Nutrition Value:

- Calories: 350 Cal
- Fat: 29 g
- Carbs: 27 g
- Protein: 15 g
- Fiber: 18 g

Lime And Avocado Tart

Preparation time: 2 hours and 40 minutes
Cooking time: 0 minutes
Servings: 8

Ingredients:

For the Crust:

- 1/4 cup shredded coconut, unsweetened
- 1/2 cup chopped pecans
- 1/2 cup chopped dates
- 2 teaspoons lime zest
- 1/8 teaspoon sea salt

For the Tart Filling:

- 1 1/2 cups avocado puree
- 1/4 cup lime juice
- 1/4 cup honey
- 1 tablespoon coconut oil
- 1 teaspoon lime zest

Method:

1. Prepare the crust, and for this, place all its ingredients in a food processor and pulse until a sticky paste comes together.
2. Spoon the mixture evenly between two mini springform pans, spread and press it evenly and then freeze for 30 minutes.
3. Meanwhile, prepare the filling, and for this, place all its ingredients in a blender and pulse until creamy.
4. Take out the frozen crusts from the freezer, pour half of the filling in one pan and the other half of filling in the second pan, smooth the top, and continue freezing for a minimum of 2 hours.
5. Then wrap each tart in plastic wrap and freeze for up to three months.
6. When ready to eat, let the tart sit at room temperature for 15 minutes, then cut it into slices and serve.

Nutrition Value:

- Calories: 224 Cal
- Fat: 14 g
- Carbs: 18 g
- Protein: 2 g
- Fiber: 4 g

Brownies

Preparation time: 15 minutes
Cooking time: 0 minutes
Servings: 8

Ingredients:

- 1 cup vanilla almonds, honey roasted
- 2 tablespoons cocoa powder
- 20 Medjool dates, pitted
- 1 tablespoon water

Method:

1. Place the almonds in a food processor, pulse until coarsely chopped, tip the almonds into a bowl and then set aside until required.
2. Add dates in the food processor, pulse until coarsely chopped, add cocoa powder and water, and pulse again until the dough comes together.
3. Add almonds, pulse again until incorporated, then transfer the dough in a large bowl and knead for 3 minutes until smooth.
4. Place a large piece of parchment paper on a clean working space, place dough on it, and roll it into 1/3-inch thick slab.
5. Use a knife to cut squares from the dough, about eight, and wrap each brownie in plastic wrap and store in the freezer for up to three months.

Nutrition Value:

- Calories: 249 Cal
- Fat: 5 g
- Carbs: 53 g
- Protein: 3 g
- Fiber: 6 g

Blueberry Custard Pie

Preparation time: 1 hour and 20 minutes
Cooking time: 8 minutes
Servings: 6

Ingredients:

For the Crust:

- 1 cup walnuts
- 2 cups dates, pitted
- 1/4 cup shredded coconut, unsweetened
- 1 cup almonds

For the Filling:

- 3 tablespoons cornstarch
- 2/3 cup coconut sugar
- 1 teaspoon vanilla extract, unsweetened
- 1 tablespoon coconut oil
- 2 cups vanilla Almond Breeze, unsweetened

For the Topping:

- 2 tablespoons blueberry jam
- 1 1/2 cups fresh blueberries

Method:

1. Prepare the crust, and for this, place all its ingredients in a food processor and pulse until ground.
2. Take a 9 inches round pan with a removable bottom, grease it with oil, spoon in crust mixture, and then spread and press it evenly into the pan, set aside until required.
3. Prepare the filling and for this, take a pot, add cornstarch and coconut sugar, stir in mixed and then whisk in the almond breeze until combined.
4. Place the pot over medium-high heat, bring the mixture to boil, then reduce heat to low level and cook for 5 minutes until the mixture has thickened, whisking continuously.
5. Remove the pot from heat, whisk in vanilla and oil until combined, then pour the filling into the crust, smooth the top and let cool.
6. Then wrap the pan tightly with a plastic wrap, refrigerate for 1 hour, and then store in the freezer for up to three months.
7. When ready to eat, let the pie rest for 20 minutes at room temperature, then cut out a slice, top it with blueberry jam and blueberries and serve.

Nutrition Value:

- Calories: 292 Cal
- Fat: 12 g
- Carbs: 44.6 g
- Protein: 3 g
- Fiber: 2.5 g

Matcha Coconut Tarts

Preparation time: 20 minutes
Cooking time: 26 minutes
Servings: 2

Ingredients:

For the Crust:

- ¼ cup shredded coconut, unsweetened
- ½ cup oat flour
- ½ cup buckwheat flour
- 4 teaspoons tapioca starch
- 1/8 teaspoon salt
- 3 tablespoons maple syrup
- 2 tablespoons cacao powder
- 3 tablespoons melted coconut oil

For the Filling:

- ½ cup cashews, soaked
- ½ teaspoon agar powder
- 2 teaspoons matcha powder
- ¼ cup maple syrup
- 1 cup coconut cream
- ¼ cup water

Method:

1. Switch on the oven, then set it to 345 degrees F, and let it preheat.
2. Meanwhile, prepare the crust, and for this, place oats in a food processor along with coconut and pulse until ground.
3. Tip the mixture in a large bowl, add buckwheat flour, cacao, salt, and tapioca starch, stir well until mixed, then gradually mix oil and maple syrup using your fingers until dough comes together, set aside for 10 minutes.
4. Then take two ramekins, grease them with oil, and line the bottom with baking paper.
5. Divide the prepared dough into two portions, place each portion in a ramekin, spread and press it in the base and sides of ramekin and bake for 16 minutes on the middle shelf of oven, let them cool completely.
6. Meanwhile, prepare the filling and for this, place cashews in a food processor, add maple syrup, matcha, and coconut cream and blend until smooth.
7. Take a small pot, place it over medium heat, pour in water, stir in agar powder, bring the mixture to boil, then switch heat to medium-low level and simmer for 15 minutes until agar has dissolved, let the mixture cool for 10 minutes.
8. Pour the agar mixture into the food processor and pulse for 1 minute until smooth.

9. Evenly divide the filling between two ramekins, smooth the top and refrigerate for 30 minutes until tarts have set.
10. Wrap each tart in plastic wrap and store in the refrigerator for up to five days or freeze for up to one month.

Nutrition Value:

- Calories: 260 Cal
- Fat: 13 g
- Carbs: 31 g
- Protein: 3 g
- Fiber: 5 g

Chocolate Chia Pudding

Preparation time: 25 minutes
Cooking time: 0 minutes
Servings: 1

Ingredients:

- 2 tablespoons chia seeds
- 1 tablespoon cacao powder
- 1/2 teaspoon vanilla extract, unsweetened
- 1 tablespoon maple syrup
- 1/2 cup milk
- Fresh strawberries as needed for topping
- Shredded coconut as needed for topping

Method:

1. Take a small glass jar, place chia seeds in it, ass cocoa powder, pour in milk, stir well and let it rest for 15 minutes.
2. Stir the chia seeds again, then stir in vanilla and maple syrup and top with strawberries and coconut.
3. Tighten the jar with the lid and store the pudding in the refrigerator for up to three days or freeze for up to one month.

Nutrition Value:

- Calories: 191 Cal
- Fat: 11 g
- Carbs: 16 g
- Protein: 8 g
- Fiber: 8 g

Rice Crispy Treats

Preparation time: 1 hour and 10 minutes
Cooking time: 0 minutes
Servings: 12

Ingredients:

- 4 cups brown rice crisp cereal
- 2 tablespoons chocolate chips
- ⅔ cup brown rice syrup
- 1/8 teaspoon salt
- 1/2 teaspoon vanilla extract, unsweetened
- 1 tablespoon coconut oil
- 1/4 cup almond butter

Method:

1. Place the brown rice cereal in a large bowl and set aside until required.
2. Take a saucepan, place it over medium heat, add oil, butter, and brown rice syrup, stir well and cook for 5 minutes until creamy.
3. Remove the pan from heat, whisk in salt and vanilla, then pour the mixture over cereal and stir until well combined.
4. Take a square baking dish, line it with parchment paper, transfer prepared cereal on it, and spread and press in the base by using your hands.
5. Top the cereal with chocolate chips, press into the cereal, and refrigerate for 1 hour.
6. Then cut the cereal into squares, wrap each square in plastic wrap and store in refrigerator for up to one week or freeze for up to two months.

Nutrition Value:

- Calories: 161 Cal
- Fat: 5 g
- Carbs: 27 g
- Protein: 2 g
- Fiber: 1 g

Conclusion

This e-book can save you with the hassle of doing a month-long meal prepping with its delicious and simple recipes. The recipes are pretty simple and easy to stick to your gluten-free diet. And, they deliver overall fantastic health benefits. You can even swap ingredients with your favorite ones and experiment with the recipes to make your meal plan that you will look forward to eating all month long.

Indeed, meal prepping makes cooking so much easy, simple, and healthy in today's busy life.

CPSIA information can be obtained
at www.ICGtesting.com
Printed in the USA
BVHW090211201222
654618BV00020B/186